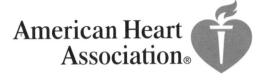

American Heart
Association®

Fighting Heart Disease and Stroke

Heartsaver AED
for the Lay Rescuer and First Responder

ADULT CARDIOPULMONARY RESUSCITATION AND AUTOMATED EXTERNAL DEFIBRILLATION

Editors

Tom P. Aufderheide, MD
Edward R. Stapleton, EMT-P
Mary Fran Hazinski, RN, MSN

Senior Science Editor

Richard O. Cummins, MD, MPH, MSc

ISBN 0-87493-690-X

Subcommittee on Basic Life Support, 1997-1998

Tom P. Aufderheide, MD, Chair

Lance B. Becker, MD, Immediate Past Chair

Thomas A. Barnes, EdD, RRT

Robert A. Berg, MD

Nisha C. Chandra, MD

Ahamed H. Idris, MD

L. Murray Lorance, EMT-D

Keith Lurie, MD

Graham Nichol, MD, MPH

James W. Parham, Jr, MA, RN

Paul E. Pepe, MD, MPH

Edward R. Stapleton, EMT-P

Wanchun Tang, MD

Terence D. Valenzuela, MD

Special Contributors

Alidene M. Doherty, RN; Anita Bailey, NREMT-P;
Terence D. Valenzuela, MD; Stacey Baker;
L. Murray Lorance, EMT-D; Jim Scappini, EMT-D;
Ronald W. Quinsey; William H. Montgomery, MD;
AHA volunteers of Florida and Texas who participated in
pilot evaluations of the Heartsaver AED Course;
AHA ECC Subcommittees on Advanced Cardiac Life Support,
Pediatric Resuscitation, and Program Administration 1997-1998

Reviewers

Donald Gordon, PhD, MD

Jo Haag, RN

Joanne L. Hirsch

Peter Kudenchuk, MD

Mary E. Mancini, RN, MSN

Eric Niegelberg, EMT-P

Greg Wayrich, EMT-P

John L. Zirkle

CONTENTS

On August 15, 2000, the AHA released the new *Guidelines 2000 for Cardiopulmonary Resuscitation and Emergency Cardiovascular Care: International Consensus on Science.* These evidence-based science guidelines recommended several changes in the teaching and practice of BLS for lay rescuers to simplify the steps and increase the effectiveness of CPR. This page and the next summarize those changes.

When the AHA revises the Heartsaver AED Course materials in 2001, all new science changes will be incorporated into all the course materials. Until the release of the revised materials the instructor should reproduce these 2 pages, and participants should insert them into their course manuals and use these pages to correct their manual. General changes in science are provided below, followed by a list of the pages in the student manual where changes should be made to reflect the new recommendations.

MAJOR CHANGES IN CPR RECOMMENDATIONS

■ **For the adult victim the lay rescuer should provide rescue breaths over 2 seconds rather than over 1½ to 2 seconds.** This slower delivery of rescue breaths should ensure that the breaths enter the victim's lungs rather than the stomach.

■ **The lay rescuer no longer checks for a pulse to determine if chest compressions and use of an AED are required.** New science has documented that the pulse is a very unreliable indicator of the presence or absence of cardiac arrest and that rescuer attempts to locate a pulse may delay the performance of chest compressions. **The rescuer should look for "signs of circulation" rather than a pulse to determine if chest compressions and use of an AED are required.** The absence of signs of circulation is one of the signs of cardiac arrest, and the rescuer should perform chest compressions and attach an AED when signs of circulation are absent. When reviewing the student manual or observing videos, participants should replace *check for a pulse* with *signs of circulation* in every instance.

Signs of circulation include a check for *normal breathing, coughing, or movement.* To check for signs of circulation you should place your ear next to the victim's mouth and nose and look, listen, and feel for normal breathing or coughing. Then quickly scan the victim to check for movement. If the victim is not breathing normally, not coughing, and not moving, you should perform chest compressions or use the AED as instructed in the manual or video.

■ **The new rate for chest compressions should be approximately 100 compressions per minute rather than 80 to 100 compressions per minute.** New science supports a faster compression rate to achieve optimal circulation during the performance of CPR.

■ **The new ratio for chest compressions during 2-rescuer CPR should be 15 compressions to 2 breaths for 1 or 2 rescuers.** New science supports longer episodes of compressions to achieve optimal circulation during the performance of CPR.

■ **New science supports simplification of the approach to lay rescuer management of foreign-body airway obstruction in the unresponsive victim.** If the lay rescuer encounters a responsive victim of FBAO who becomes unresponsive or if the rescuer suspects an airway obstruction in an unresponsive victim, the lay rescuer should perform CPR. Each time the airway is opened, the rescuer looks for an obstructing object in the back of the throat. If the rescuer sees an object, she or he should remove it. This simplification should improve the learning and retention of core CPR skills.

PAGES IN PARTICIPANT MANUAL ON WHICH TO MAKE SCIENCE CHANGES

Participants may wish to make corrections in this manual to reflect the 2000 science changes.

Science Changes	Manual Page	Suggested Revision
Simplification of procedure for managing an unconscious victim of foreign-body airway obstruction	1-12, 2-11, 2-12, 2-13	**Replace the complete procedure for the unresponsive/ unconscious FBAO victim with the following:** If a responsive/conscious victim of FBAO becomes unresponsive/unconscious or if you encounter an unsuspected airway obstruction in an unresponsive victim, perform CPR. After attempting and reattempting ventilation during the performance of CPR, continue the sequence of chest compressions and ventilations. Each time the airway is opened, look for an obstructing object in the back of the throat. If you see an object, remove it.
Increased time for delivery of rescue breaths for adult victims	2-6 (box), A-8, C-5	**Replace rescue breaths taking 1½ to 2 seconds with breaths that take longer:** Give 2 slow breaths (take 2 seconds for each breath).
Signs of cardiac arrest in adults: Unresponsiveness and breathlessness are still valid signs of cardiac arrest. However, "pulse" is replaced with "signs of circulation."	1-9, 1-10, 2-5* (*change occurs several times), 2-6, 2-7*, 2-14*, 2-15*, 3-6, 3-10*, 3-11, 4-1*, 4-3*, 4-4*, 4-9*, 4-10*, 4-11*, 4-14*, 4-19*, 4-20*, 6-4, 6-5*, 6-8, A-8*, B-3, C-1, C-4*, C-5, D-5, E-3, E-4*, E-6*	Replace "no pulse" with "no signs of circulation (no normal breathing, coughing, or movement in response to the 2 rescue breaths)." Replace "pulse" or "pulse present" with "signs of circulation" or "signs of circulation present."
All references to checking for a pulse (for adult and pediatric victims) should be changed to checking for signs of circulation (normal breathing, coughing, or movement)	2-3, 2-5*, 2-7*, 2-15*, 2-6*, 3-1, 3-9*, 3-10*, 3-12, 4-5, 4-9*, 4-10*, 4-14, A-8, E-3, E-4*, E-5, E-6*	Whenever the text instructs rescuers to "check for a pulse," lay rescuers should substitute "check for signs of circulation (normal breathing, coughing, or movement)."
Increased rate of chest compression for adult victims	2-7	Replace compress "at a rate of 80 to 100" with "at a rate of approximately 100 per minute."
Compression-ventilation ratio for 2-rescuer CPR	2-9	The ratio for 2-rescuer CPR is 15 compressions to 2 ventilations (same as 1-rescuer CPR).
Skills performance sheet	A-8	In HS-AED skills performance sheet, substitute "check for signs of circulation (normal breathing, coughing, movement)" for "check for pulse" and "check for carotid pulse" as an indication to begin chest compressions and attach the AED for performance criteria and critical actions.

INTRODUCTION

You can save the life of a loved one, a friend, a coworker, or a citizen in your community with the skills you learn in the American Heart Association's Heartsaver AED Course. The AHA developed and tested this course in 1997-1998 to support the growing movement toward **public access defibrillation.** In public access defibrillation, or "witness defibrillation," the person who sees someone in cardiac arrest gives the victim defibrillation shocks. The "witness" is most often a lay rescuer, perhaps the victim's friend or coworker. The **automated external defibrillator (AED)** is a new and important device used in emergency cardiovascular care. AEDs are accurate, easy to operate, and have saved many lives. They can be used effectively by laypeople with minimal training.

You may work in a place where someone has decided to start a public access defibrillation program. More and more people like you who are trained in cardiopulmonary resuscitation (CPR) also need to learn how to use AEDs. In many communities AEDs can be used by firefighters, police, security guards, commercial airline crews, trained laypersons, and family members of cardiac patients who are at high risk for cardiac arrest. Both **early CPR** and **early defibrillation** — two links in what we call the **Chain of Survival** — save lives. Getting the defibrillator — and someone who can operate it — to a collapsed person in a few short minutes is the first step in achieving early defibrillation and saving a life.

The Heartsaver AED Course teaches the basic techniques of adult CPR and use of an AED. You will also learn about using barrier devices in CPR and giving first aid for choking. This

As a Heartsaver trained in CPR and use of an AED, you may help save a life.

course follows the AHA guidelines for performing CPR and using an AED. These are integrated skills that you can learn best in one 3½- to 4-hour course. Some of you will be taking this course for general information because an AED is not available where you live or work. Others will be given specific training on the AED available at your home or worksite. The course instructor may adjust some details of CPR and AED operation to fit your particular setting and the brand of AED you will use.

These are the major **knowledge objectives** (cognitive objectives) of the course:

1. Describe the links in the AHA Chain of Survival.
2. Describe how to activate the local emergency medical services (EMS) system.
3. Recognize the signs of 4 major emergencies:
   a. Heart attack
   b. Cardiac arrest
   c. Stroke
   d. Foreign-body airway obstruction

These are the major **skills objectives** (psychomotor objectives) of the course:

1. Demonstrate the following skills of the Heartsaver AED rescuer using an adult manikin, an AED (or suitable trainer model), pocket face mask, and telephone:
   a. Calling 911 and getting the AED
   b. Rescue breathing using mouth-to-mouth and mouth-to–face mask techniques
   c. One-rescuer adult CPR
   d. Relief of adult foreign-body airway obstruction
   e. Safe defibrillation with an AED in less than 90 seconds of AED placement at the training manikin's side (less than 90 seconds is the maximum acceptable time)
2. Demonstrate how to troubleshoot the most common problems you might encounter while using an AED.

This course handbook contains several features designed to help you learn the essential skills of CPR and AED operation.

These features include learning objectives, review questions, and skills review sheets. These will help make learning easier and more complete. At the start of each chapter, carefully read the learning objectives. They will help you focus on essential information before you read the chapter. When you have finished reading the chapter, answer the review questions. If you cannot answer a question or if you choose the wrong answer, review the parts of the chapter related to that question.

The skills sheets ("Performance Criteria") in appendix A present the CPR and AED skills you will practice in class. Review each skill, pay attention to the details, and practice carefully. You can forget many simple skills, so remember to practice from time to time after the course. The course instructor will tell you how often to practice and the best way to practice. This handbook will be a valuable resource for you before, during, and after your training.

Public access defibrillation using AEDs is a new and dynamic field. In most states public access defibrillation is so new that legislators must revise state laws and regulations to allow defibrillation by nonprofessionals or Good Samaritans. The information in the AHA Heartsaver AED Course will change over time. The AHA will continue to reevaluate the guidelines for CPR and automated external defibrillation and revise them when necessary. We encourage you to stay informed about changes in basic life support (BLS) and CPR techniques. The AHA newsletter *Currents in Emergency Cardiovascular Care* is an excellent source of up-to-date information.

We wish you success as you learn the skills of CPR and early defibrillation. When you complete the course, you will be better prepared to face future emergencies with powerful tools and effective skills.

AEDs are accurate, easy to operate, and have saved many lives.

CONTENTS

LEARNING OBJECTIVES

1. Name the links in the AHA adult Chain of Survival and discuss the role you play in the chain.
2. List the signs of these 4 major emergencies:
   a. Heart attack
   b. Cardiac arrest
   c. Stroke
   d. Airway obstruction by a foreign body (conscious choking)

STUDY QUESTIONS

As you read this chapter, try to answer these questions:

Chain of Survival

1. There are 4 links in the AHA Chain of Survival. What are they?
2. In the Heartsaver AED Course you are learning to perform the critical actions that compose 3 of the 4 links in the Chain of Survival. What are they?
3. Why is it important that *you* defibrillate with an AED rather than wait for emergency rescuers who are better trained than you are?

Heart Attack

1. How do people who are having a heart attack usually describe the pain?
2. Where is this pain usually located?
3. How long does the pain of a heart attack usually last?

Cardiac Arrest

1. There are 3 major signs of a cardiac arrest. What are they?

Stroke

1. How is the headache caused by a stroke often described?
2. What abnormalities may you see in facial muscles, arm movement, and speech in a person with stroke?
3. When should you activate the EMS system if you think someone has had a stroke?

Foreign-Body Airway Obstruction (Conscious Choking)

1. What is the universal sign that a person who cannot speak may use to indicate that he or she is choking?
2. A choking person says, "Help me! I'm choking!" How do you help him or her?
3. A person who is choking falls to the floor unconscious. How do you treat this person?

Every year 225,000 adult Americans die from cardiac arrest.

. . . .

When you recognize an emergency, the first three links in the Chain of Survival are in **your** *hands.* **You** *call 911.* **You** *begin CPR.* **You** *use the AED.*

. . . .

Cardiovascular disease is the single greatest cause of death in the United States. Every year more than 480,000 adult Americans die of a **heart attack** or its complications. About half (250,000) of these deaths result from **sudden cardiac arrest,** a complication of heart attack. A cardiac arrest can occur within seconds of the heart attack, before the victim arrives at the hospital. It will result in death unless immediate emergency treatment is provided.

The victim of an emergency such as a heart attack, cardiac arrest, stroke, or foreign-body airway obstruction can be saved if people at the scene act quickly to start the **Chain of Survival.** In this chapter you will learn the critical actions that compose 4 links in the AHA Chain of Survival. You will learn how to recognize the symptoms of a heart attack, cardiac arrest, stroke, and foreign-body airway obstruction (choking) and when to call 911.

One link in the Chain of Survival is **cardiopulmonary resuscitation, or CPR.** With CPR you provide oxygen-rich blood to the brain and heart until defibrillation and more advanced care can be given.

Another link in the Chain of Survival is **defibrillation.** Defibrillation delivers an electric current ("shock") to the heart to stop abnormal electric activity. This allows the heart to resume normal function. You will learn to provide defibrillation using an **automated external defibrillator (AED).** An AED is a device that evaluates the patient's heart rhythm, generates and delivers an electric charge, and reevaluates the heart rhythm. All AEDs provide both voice and visual prompts to lead you through important rescue steps.

THE AHA CHAIN OF SURVIVAL SYMBOL

The AHA Chain of Survival symbol (FIGURE 1) depicts the critical actions required to treat any life-threatening emergency, including heart attack, cardiac arrest, stroke, and airway obstruction by a foreign body.

Once you recognize an emergency, you should *immediately*

- **Call 911** to activate the emergency medical services (EMS) system and send someone to get the AED.
- **Begin CPR.**
- **Use the AED.**
- **Transfer to advanced care** (when skilled EMS rescuers arrive).

You must know when to activate the Chain of Survival. You must recognize that an emergency exists. When you recognize the emergency, the first 3 links — call 911, begin CPR, and use the AED — are in your hands. *You* perform these actions. *You* connect the links that increase a person's chance of survival. Skilled emergency professionals will respond to the 911 call. You can then transfer the person to them for advanced care.

To save people with heart attack, cardiac arrest, or stroke, *each set of actions or link in the Chain of Survival must be performed as soon as possible.* If any link in the chain is weak, delayed, or missing, the chances of survival are lessened.

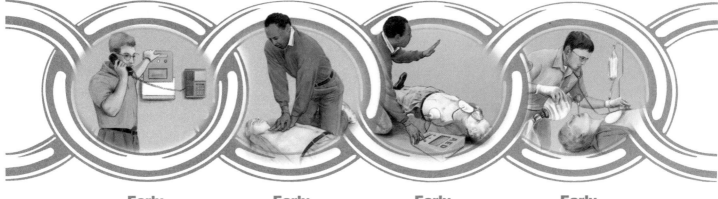

| Early Access | Early CPR | Early Defibrillation | Early Advanced Care |

FIGURE 1.
The AHA Chain of Survival. The 4 links or actions in the chain are (1) call 911 and get the AED, (2) begin CPR, (3) use the AED, and (4) transfer to advanced care.

Unresponsiveness

is a red flag

for an

emergency —

you need to act

immediately!

THE LINKS IN THE CHAIN OF SURVIVAL

Recognize an Emergency

First, you or other witnesses must recognize the emergency. You must recognize the warning signs of a heart attack, cardiac arrest, stroke, or choking. *Anyone* who is *unresponsive* should receive emergency care. Heart attack, cardiac arrest, stroke, and foreign-body airway obstruction can each cause unresponsiveness. Although many conditions — not just cardiac arrest — can cause unresponsiveness, *all* unresponsive victims will benefit from activation of the Chain of Survival.

Call 911 (or the EMS System in Your Area) and Get the AED

As soon as an emergency is recognized, call 911. Keep the AED near the telephone in the home, worksite, or public building. The person who calls 911 can return with the AED.

When you or another rescuer calls 911, let the dispatcher ask you questions. While the dispatcher interviews you, he or she will enter the data on a computer. The information you give will be relayed to a response team. Answer in short, specific replies, giving only the requested information. The dispatcher will probably ask

- **"What is your emergency?"** You might answer, *"A customer had sudden chest pain and has now collapsed."*
- **"What's happening now?"** *"My friend is giving CPR! We have an AED."*
- **"Where is the patient located?"** *"We are at the Evergreen Company, here at 1234 Fifth Avenue NE, in the back hall."*
- **"What number are you calling from?"** *"The number is 555-1313."*

At this point the dispatcher may give you directions such as, **"Stay on the line until I tell you to hang up. Rescuers are being sent to your location. Please meet them and direct them to the scene."**

Dispatcher-Assisted CPR and Defibrillation and Enhanced 911

In many areas of country emergency dispatchers are taught how to help callers give emergency care. With help from the dispatcher, callers can give CPR and use an AED. The instructions are basic and simple, but they will help the victim until EMS personnel arrive. Remember, early CPR and early defibrillation are critical links in the Chain of Survival and need to be started immediately.

Using a prepared list of instructions, the dispatcher can coach you through the basic steps of CPR and use of your AED. At a worksite you will usually have help. Use this approach:

- Repeat the dispatcher's instructions loudly to the other rescuers and confirm that they are following that step.

- If the patient vomits or other complications arise, tell the dispatcher. Do not expect that you will perform perfectly in such a crisis.

- Be sure that rescuers follow each instruction, even if it takes extra seconds.

- Ensure rescuer safety at all times.

- When EMS personnel arrive at the victim's side, the dispatcher will tell you that he or she is hanging up.

- You hang up last.

Public access defibrillation programs and AED manufacturers should work with local EMS systems. Program authorities or manufacturers should notify EMS directors of AEDs placed in homes, businesses, or other public areas.

Find out if your community has *enhanced 911*. In enhanced 911 a computer automatically confirms the caller's address. Also ask if your 911 dispatchers are trained to offer pre-arrival instructions to rescuers. This means that they can give instructions for immediate care based on the clinical *criteria* of the emergency. If not, become a vocal advocate for such services in your community. Enhanced 911 can save precious seconds, minutes, and even lives.

Begin Cardiopulmonary Resuscitation

CPR is the critical link that buys time between the first link (call 911) and the third link (use the AED). The earlier you give CPR to a person in cardiac or respiratory arrest, the greater their chance of survival. CPR keeps oxygenated blood flowing to the brain and heart until defibrillation or other advanced care can restore normal heart action.

Use the Automated External Defibrillator to Treat Ventricular Fibrillation

Most sudden cardiac arrest victims are in **ventricular fibrillation (VF).** VF is an abnormal, chaotic heart rhythm that prevents the heart from pumping blood. VF causes more cardiac arrests than any other rhythm.

You must defibrillate a victim immediately to stop VF and allow a normal heart rhythm to resume. The sooner you provide defibrillation with the AED, the better the victim's chances of

PUBLIC ACCESS DEFIBRILLATION

The AHA promotes the most rapid possible defibrillation of victims of cardiac arrest. To do this the AHA wants to place AEDs in the hands of trained, nontraditional rescuers. These include police, security guards, and family members of patients at high risk for cardiac arrest.

Public access defibrillation (PAD) programs place AEDs in homes, police cars, worksites, and public gathering places, under the supervision of licensed physicians. PAD rescuers must be trained in CPR and use of an AED. When AEDs are readily available, rescuers can provide defibrillation within the first few minutes of out-of-hospital cardiac arrest. This dramatically increases the victim's chances of survival.

The AHA has developed the Heartsaver AED Course to support the PAD movement and specific PAD programs. The course is designed to help you learn how to give CPR and use an AED. These skills are essential in caring for the victim of cardiac arrest.

- As a Heartsaver trained in both CPR and use of an AED, you can increase the chances of survival for a victim of cardiac arrest. You may help save a life.

- The most frequent cause of cardiac arrest is the sudden onset of the deadly rhythm VF.

- You can keep the heart and brain alive by performing CPR while you wait for the AED to arrive.

- The only effective treatment for VF is electric defibrillation with a defibrillator.

- The sooner you perform defibrillation, the greater the chance that defibrillation will work.

- The Heartsaver AED Course enables you to perform the life-saving skills of CPR and use of an AED for victims of cardiac arrest.

survival. If you provide defibrillation within the first 5 minutes of a cardiac arrest, the odds are about 50% that you can save the victim's life. But with each passing minute during a cardiac arrest, the chance of successful resuscitation is reduced by 7% to 10%. After 10 minutes there is very little chance of successful rescue.

Transfer to Advanced Care

The fourth link in the Chain of Survival is advanced care. This link is provided by highly trained EMS personnel called "paramedics." Paramedics give CPR and defibrillation as well as more advanced care. They can give cardiac drugs and insert endotracheal breathing tubes. These advanced actions (1) help the heart in VF respond to defibrillation or (2) maintain a normal rhythm after successful defibrillation.

HOW TO RECOGNIZE MAJOR EMERGENCIES:

HEART ATTACK, CARDIAC ARREST, STROKE, AND FOREIGN-BODY AIRWAY OBSTRUCTION (CHOKING)

How to Recognize a Heart Attack

A heart attack means some heart muscle has suddenly started to die. The muscle is dying because one of the heart's major blood vessels (a coronary artery) has become blocked. The artery can be blocked by buildup of cholesterol deposits or by a blood clot. *Acute myocardial infarction* is the medical term for heart attack.

A person having a heart attack is usually awake and can talk to you but feels severe pain. The most critical time for treatment of heart attack is the first 30 minutes after symptoms begin. If you suspect someone is having a heart attack, activate the EMS system immediately. These minutes count! Know the symptoms!

The most important and most common symptom of a heart attack is chest pain or pressure in the center of the chest, behind the breastbone (sternum). The pain lasts more than 3 to 5 minutes. Consider **chest pain** *a red flag. The flag says Warning! You should think of a heart attack.*

You can ask these questions:

- "*What* is the pain like?" People describe the pain of a heart attack in many ways: a "pressure," "fullness," "squeezing," or "heaviness."

- "*Where* is the pain located?" Usually people feel the pain right behind the breastbone, deep in the center of the chest (**FIGURE 2**). After a few moments the pain may seem to spread to the shoulder, the neck, the lower jaw, or down the arm. The pain may be on the left side or the right side or on both sides. Sometimes the pain or discomfort may even be felt in the back, between the shoulder blades.

- "*How long* does the pain last?" The discomfort of a heart attack usually lasts more than a few minutes. Sharp, stabbing, knifelike pain that lasts only a second and then disappears is almost never heart attack pain. Heart attack chest pain sometimes "stutters." This means the pain may stop completely but returns a short time later.

Many people will not admit that their symptoms may indicate a heart attack. People react with a variety of statements or excuses. They may say "I'm too healthy" or "I don't want to bother the doctor" or "I don't want to frighten my wife" or "I'll feel ridiculous if it isn't a heart attack" or "I hate red lights and sirens."

When a person with symptoms of a heart attack tries to downplay what he or she is feeling, **you** must take responsibility and act at once. Tell the victim to sit quietly. Tell the nearest person to call 911 and get the AED. Be prepared to perform CPR if necessary.

After you or someone else calls 911, have the person rest quietly and calmly. Help the person into a position that is the most comfortable and that allows the easiest breathing.

How to Recognize a Cardiac Arrest

When blocked arteries deprive the heart muscle of oxygen during a heart attack, the heart may actually stop beating. This produces a **cardiac arrest:** no blood flow and no pulse. Without blood flow to the brain, the person becomes unconscious, collapses, and stops breathing normally. Often VF stops the rhythmic contractions of the heart. VF leads to chaotic, quivering, and uncoordinated spasms of the heart muscle.

VF starts in the same damaged areas of the heart muscle that produce the severe chest pain of a heart attack. VF can begin in mildly damaged areas of the heart, even in men or women without chest pain. Sudden VF and cardiac arrest may be the only sign of a heart attack in some victims. The only treatment for VF is electrical shocks from a defibrillator.

It is critical for you to recognize that an unresponsive person may be in cardiac arrest. Unresponsiveness is a red flag for an emergency — you need to act immediately!

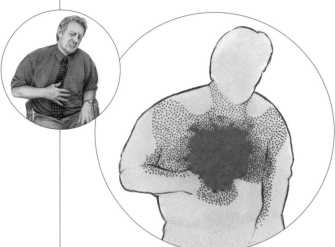

FIGURE 2.
Typical locations of chest pain in persons having a heart attack.

FOUNDATION FACTS: WARNING SIGNS AND SYMPTOMS

Not *all* warning symptoms occur in *every* heart attack. If any occur, don't wait. Get help immediately. Call 911. Delay can be deadly! People who are having a heart attack may complain of signs or symptoms other than chest pain. These additional red flags, or warning symptoms, of a heart attack include

- *Lightheadedness*, "feeling dizzy" during the pain
- *Fainting*, completely losing consciousness, especially when the pain starts
- *Sweating*, breaking out in a "cold sweat all over" but without a fever
- *Nausea*, usually without vomiting — "I feel sick"
- *Shortness of breath*, especially worrisome if the victim is short of breath during pain, while lying still or resting, or when moving only a little

1. *Unresponsiveness:* The person is unconscious and does not respond when you call their name or touch them. At this point tell someone to activate the EMS system and get the AED.

2. *Breathlessness:* The person does not take a normal breath when you check for several seconds. You discover that the person is breathless only after you begin the sequence of CPR: open the airway and look, listen, and feel for respirations.

3. *Pulselessness:* You feel no pulse in the person's neck. You confirm that the person is pulseless only after you have delivered 2 breaths to the breathless victim.

How to Recognize a Stroke

Stroke happens fast. Stroke is the rapid onset of neurological problems like weakness, paralysis in one or more limbs (particularly the hand), difficulties with speaking, visual problems, intense dizziness, facial weakness, altered consciousness, or severe headache. Stroke occurs when one of two events happen in the brain: (1) a blood vessel is blocked by a blood clot so that an area of the brain receives no blood flow and no oxygen or (2) a blood vessel breaks open and blood pours out into or over the brain. Strokes are common, serious, and often sudden. *Stroke is a leading cause of death and serious disability among Americans.*

Strokes sometimes cause such severe brain damage that the victim stops breathing or develops a blocked airway. You may need to perform some or all of the steps of CPR: rescue breathing, chest compressions, or both. Although most strokes occur in older people, *strokes can happen in persons of all ages.*

You should know the *red flags* or **signs of stroke** so that you can activate the EMS system. Signs of stroke range from very mild signs to loss of consciousness and coma. The most common complaints include the following:

- Severe headache (often described as "the worst headache of my life")

- Visual disturbances such as blurring or double vision

- Slurring or loss of speech or incoherent speech

- Loss of movement, weakness, unsteadiness, or falls

- Dizziness or nausea

Unfortunately many of the signs of stroke can be vague or ignored by the victim. If you are concerned that someone has had a stroke, look closely for one of the following 3 signs:

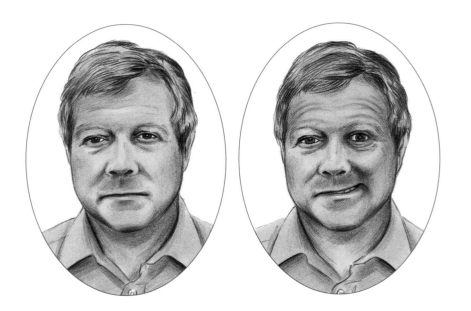

FIGURE 3.
Stroke patient with facial droop (right side of the patient's face). Left, Patient in repose. Right, After the command, "Look up and smile showing all your teeth."

1. **Facial droop:** This is most obvious if the victim smiles or grimaces. If one side of the face droops or the face does not move **(FIGURE 3),** a stroke may have occurred.

2. **Arm weakness:** This is most obvious if the victim extends his or her arms with eyes closed. If one arm drifts downward or the arms can't move, this may indicate a stroke.

3. **Speech difficulties:** This is most obvious if the victim is unable to speak or slurs words. Ask the victim to repeat a sentence such as "You can't teach an old dog new tricks." If the victim cannot repeat the phrase or sentence accurately and clearly, a stroke may have occurred.

Whenever you see signs of stroke, call 911. EMS personnel will examine the person and transport him or her to a hospital for evaluation and treatment. Wonderful new treatments for stroke are now available. These include "clot busters" for the brain (thrombolytic agents), which may reduce or eliminate brain damage from a stroke. These treatments, however, must be given within minutes of the onset of stroke. To help treat a stroke victim, bystanders and lay rescuers must

- Recognize the signs of stroke.
- Call 911.
- Provide CPR if needed.
- Transfer the victim to trained EMS personnel for rapid transport to the emergency department.

CRITICAL CONCEPTS:
RED-FLAG SIGNS OF SEVERE FOREIGN-BODY AIRWAY OBSTRUCTION

- The *"universal choking signal"* (clutching the neck with one or both hands) **(FIGURE 4)**
- Poor, ineffective coughs
- Inability to speak
- High-pitched sounds while inhaling
- Increased difficulty breathing
- Blue lips or skin (cyanosis)
- Loss of consciousness and responsiveness

Do not make the mistake of thinking that a stroke victim's symptoms are caused by alcohol or drug intoxication or medical conditions such as low blood sugar. If you suspect that a person is having a stroke, call 911 at once.

How to Recognize Airway Obstruction by a Foreign Body (Choking)

Every year airway obstruction by foreign bodies or choking causes about 3185 deaths. Foreign-body obstruction of the airway in the adult usually occurs during eating. Meat is the most frequent cause of choking in adults, but a variety of foods and foreign bodies have caused airway obstruction in children and some adults.

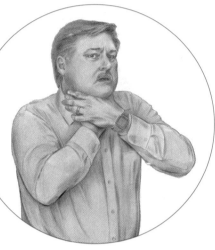

FIGURE 4.
Universal choking signal.

To treat airway obstruction successfully, **you must recognize it.** For all choking victims, if a foreign body is obstructing the airway it must be removed. Otherwise breathing or rescue breathing won't work. For conscious choking victims you help clear the airway. For unconscious choking victims you open the airway and forcefully remove the blocking object either by the Heimlich maneuver or by using your fingers.

SUMMARY

To rescue someone, you must first recognize that the person is having an emergency. The Chain of Survival for heart attack, cardiac arrest, stroke, and foreign-body airway obstruction starts with an alert fellow citizen who recognizes the emergency and takes action. This is an important step and one that will be practiced over and over again in this course.

This course encourages each participant to become a part of the community's Chain of Survival:

- Learn to recognize the 4 conditions that are major killers in the United States: heart attack, cardiac arrest, stroke, and foreign-body airway obstruction.
- Know to call 911 and activate the EMS system for these emergencies.
- Know how to open or clear an obstructed airway.
- Know how to perform CPR.
- Know how to use an AED.

With this knowledge and these skills, you can become an effective and vital link in the community's Chain of Survival.

REVIEW QUESTIONS

1. When you find an unresponsive victim, which link in the Chain of Survival should be accomplished first?

   a. call 911

   b. begin CPR

   c. use the AED

   d. transfer to advanced care

2. Which of the following is a *red-flag* symptom of a heart attack?

   a. squeezing or crushing chest pain behind the breastbone that lasts more than a few minutes

   b. sharp, stabbing chest pain that lasts only a few seconds

   c. shortness of breath

   d. "the worst headache of my life"

3. Which of the following groups of signs or symptoms are the *red-flag* signs of cardiac arrest?

   a. facial droop, arm weakness, speech difficulties

   b. chest pain, lightheadedness, sweating, and nausea

   c. unresponsiveness, breathlessness, and pulselessness

   d. unresponsiveness, spontaneous breathing, and chest pain

4. Which of the following are *red-flag* signs and symptoms of a stroke?

   a. sudden loss of consciousness and cardiac arrest

   b. facial droop, arm weakness, and speech difficulties

   c. unresponsiveness, breathlessness, and pulselessness

   d. crushing chest pain that lasts a few minutes, nausea, and sweating

5. What are the *red-flag* signs of severe airway obstruction that require your intervention?

   a. wheezing between coughs and hoarse speech

   b. severe, forceful coughing

   c. inability to speak, breathe, or cough and blue skin or lips

   d. unresponsiveness, breathlessness, and pulselessness

HOW DID YOU DO?

1. a; **2.** a; **3.** c; **4.** b; **5.** c

CONTENTS

2

LEARNING OBJECTIVES

After reading this chapter you should be able to

1. Describe and demonstrate one-rescuer CPR

2. Describe and demonstrate how to use pocket face masks during CPR

3. Recognize when someone is choking due to a foreign-body airway obstruction

4. Describe and demonstrate how to clear the airway of a conscious or unconscious person with a foreign body blocking the airway

CPR: THE SECOND LINK IN THE CHAIN OF SURVIVAL

CPR skills include a combination of rescue breathing (blowing) and chest compressions (pumping). If you find an *unresponsive* person, send someone to **call 911** and **get the *AED*. Then you start CPR**. CPR is the second link in the Chain of Survival. Continue CPR until additional treatment (for example, defibrillation with an AED) restores normal heart action.

CPR helps the heart respond better to defibrillation shocks. For this reason it is critical to begin CPR at once. Do not wait for the AED to arrive. You will also give CPR *between* AED shocks (usually after every 3 shocks). You do this to provide oxygen to the heart and to increase the chances that defibrillation will succeed.

Check the victim: If the victim is *unresponsive*, *call 911* and *get the AED.*

NOTE: In chapters 3 and 4 you will learn how to combine CPR and defibrillation. Defibrillation provides a step "D" to go with the ABCs of CPR. Always begin with the ABCs when you find an unconscious victim. Go to step D if the victim does not have a pulse. The AED appears in the figures for this chapter but is not taught until chapters 3 and 4.

When you encounter an emergency — at home, at work, or in the community — quickly determine unresponsiveness to decide whether to call 911. Then get the AED from its location near the telephone:

1. **First, check to see if the victim is unresponsive** by gently shaking the victim and shouting, "Are you OK?" **(FIGURE 1).**

   • **If the victim does not respond,** send someone to **call 911** and **get the AED!** This activates the EMS system, ensures

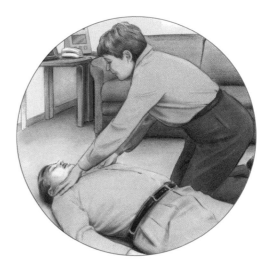

FIGURE 1.
Unresponsive.

CRITICAL CONCEPTS: UNRESPONSIVE — 911 — AED

To help you remember these first actions, think of this short phrase: Unresponsive — 911 — AED. These are critical steps you must do before the ABCs. Whether you are responding in a crowded worksite with many helpers or you are alone — what we call "the Lone Rescuer" — you still have to make sure that either you or another person takes these actions.

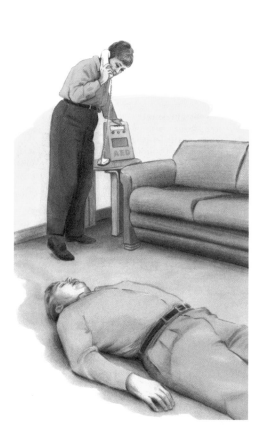

FIGURE 2.
Call 911 — get the AED.

FIGURE 3.
Airway: head tilt–chin lift.

that professional help is on the way, and brings the AED to your side in a few moments.

- **If you are alone** and find an unresponsive victim, you will have to leave the victim to call 911 and get the AED. As standard practice the AED should be stored next to a telephone. You should be able to call 911 while reaching for the AED in its carrying case (**FIGURE 2**).

- When you have sent someone to call 911 and get the AED, kneel at the victim's side near his or her head to start CPR. The victim should be on his or her back. If not, carefully turn the victim onto his or her back.

2. **Airway: open the airway with the head tilt–chin lift maneuver (FIGURE 3).**

   - Tilt the head back by lifting the chin gently with one hand while pushing down on the forehead with the other hand.

3. **Breathing: head tilt–chin lift; look, listen, and feel; 2 slow breaths:**

   To check for breathing, *look, listen, and feel:*

   a. Place your ear next to the victim's mouth and nose (**FIGURE 3**) and listen for breathing, turning your head to observe the chest.

   b. Look for the chest to rise. Listen and feel for air movement on your cheek.

   If not breathing, give 2 slow rescue breaths (FIGURE 4).
   To perform rescue breathing in the home:

   a. Place your mouth around the victim's mouth and pinch the nose closed.

   b. Continue to tilt the head and lift the chin.

   c. Give **2 slow breaths.**

   d. Be sure the victim's chest rises each time you give a rescue breath.

   To perform rescue breathing in the workplace or in a public setting:

   a. Quickly assemble the pocket face mask (available in the AED case).

   b. Place the mask over the victim's nose and mouth.

   c. Continue to tilt the head and lift the chin.

   d. Provide **2 slow breaths** into the opening of the pocket face mask.

   e. Adjust the mask as needed to ensure a tight seal. Be sure the victim's chest rises each time you blow into the mask.

4. **Circulation: Check for a pulse. If no pulse, start chest compressions.** If the victim has a pulse but is not breathing, give rescue breaths (1 breath every 5 seconds).

Ensure that someone has called *911* and is getting the *AED*.

a. Maintain head tilt.

b. Place 2 or 3 fingers on the Adam's apple (voice box). Slide the fingers into the groove between the Adam's apple and the muscle **(FIGURE 5)**.

CRITICAL CONCEPTS: AIRWAY

In CPR your first action focuses on the Airway. You *must* open the airway. Remember, the tongue is the most common cause of a blocked airway in the unconscious victim. When a victim is unconscious, the muscles of the jaw and neck relax, allowing the tongue to fall back against the throat and block the airway (FIGURE 3A).

The tongue is attached to the lower jaw, so tilting the head and lifting the chin pulls the tongue away from the back of the throat and opens the airway. Open the airway by tilting the head back and lifting the chin. This is called the *head tilt–chin lift* maneuver.

If the victim has been injured with possible head and neck trauma, open the airway with a *jaw thrust*. Grasp the angles of the victim's jaw and lift it upward without tilting the head. This method of opening the airway, the *jaw-thrust maneuver*, will also pull the tongue away from the back of the throat (FIGURE 6). The jaw thrust causes less neck movement but is a bit more difficult to perform, so it should be saved for victims with possible head or neck injuries.

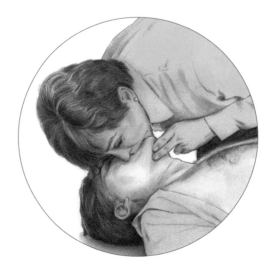

FIGURE 4.
Breathing: give 2 slow breaths.

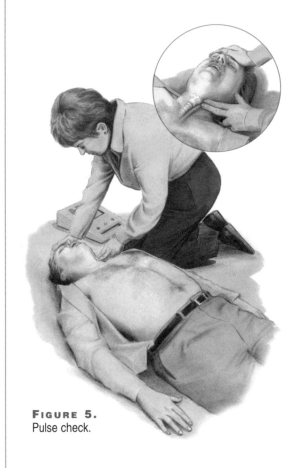

FIGURE 5.
Pulse check.

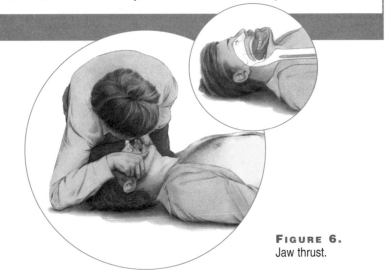

FIGURE 6.
Jaw thrust.

CRITICAL CONCEPTS: CHECK FOR THE CAROTID PULSE

Blood must circulate to deliver oxygen to the brain, heart, and other vital organs. If you can feel the pulse in the neck (the carotid artery), the victim's heart is beating adequately, and chest compressions are unnecessary. If you *cannot* feel the victim's carotid pulse within 10 seconds, then *both* chest compressions and attachment of the AED are needed.

FOUNDATION FACTS: AGONAL BREATHING

People in cardiac arrest soon stop breathing because oxygen is no longer delivered to the brain. Some victims, however, may display irregular, infrequent, gasping breaths called "agonal breaths." Agonal breaths may fool some rescuers into thinking that the victim is still alive, still responsive, and not in need of CPR or defibrillation. This could cause a missed opportunity to save a person's life.

If the victim is unconscious and pulseless, start CPR and attach the AED — even if you observe sporadic, gasping breaths. The AED can still identify the presence or absence of VF and clarify the victim's status.

FOUNDATION FACTS: WHY BREATHING?

When breathing stops, oxygen delivery to the heart and brain stops. If oxygen delivery is not restored immediately, the heart and brain may be damaged. The longer the victim is deprived of oxygen, the smaller the chance that he or she will respond to CPR. Mouth-to-mouth or mouth-to-mask breathing is the quickest way to deliver oxygen to the victim's lungs and blood.

When providing rescue breathing, check to see that the victim's chest rises with each breath you give. This is critical because it is the only way you can tell that you are giving good rescue breaths.

Breaths must be delivered slowly. Take 1½ to 2 seconds to deliver each breath. You do not want to give rapid, forceful breaths, which can blow air into the esophagus and stomach instead of the lungs. Air in the stomach can cause vomiting, which complicates CPR in many ways.

If a victim has dentures, leave them in place. Dentures help provide a good mouth-to-mouth or mouth-to-mask seal. An exception to this rule occurs when the dentures are extremely loose. Loose dentures should be removed so that they do not fall back into the throat and obstruct the airway.

When you *look, listen, and feel* for breathing and find that the victim *is breathing*, you don't need to provide the 2 rescue breaths. Watch the victim to be sure that breathing continues. If the breathing is adequate, you may place the victim on his or her side in the recovery position to keep the airway open.

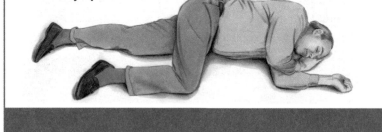

c. Feel for the pulse with your fingers for 10 seconds.

d. If no pulse, start chest compressions. Find a position on the lower half of the sternum, right between the nipples (FIGURE 7).

e. Place the heel of one hand on the *center* of the breastbone right between the nipples.

f. Place the heel of the second hand on top of the first hand.

g. Position your body directly over your hands. Your shoulders should be above your hands, and you should look down on your hands.

h. Provide 15 compressions at a rate of 80 to 100 compressions per minute (slightly faster than 1 compression per second). Your instructor will give you suggestions about ways to maintain the correct speed.

5. **"Pump and blow":* Cycles: 15 chest compressions, 2 rescue breaths.**

a. Continue one-rescuer CPR with **15** chest compressions (**"pump"**) and 2 slow breaths (**"blow"**) (FIGURE 8).

b. After 1 minute of CPR (4 cycles of 15 compressions and 2 breaths), check the pulse to see if circulation has been restored. *Check the pulse* every few minutes. If a pulse returns, stop chest compressions and continue providing rescue breaths if needed (1 breath every 5 seconds).

KEEPING YOUR SKILLS SHARP: CPR PRACTICE

Review the steps and skills of one-rescuer CPR regularly (several times every year). If you learn CPR at work, try to practice it on a manikin with coworkers. If you learn CPR for a loved one at home, review practice videos and CPR prompt devices that use recorded instructions. Renew your CPR skills with an instructor at least every 2 years by taking an AHA refresher course.

The Heartsaver AED Course teaches you the skills of adult CPR. Other AHA courses add instruction on CPR, treatment of choking in infants and children, and other skills.

Never rehearse or practice CPR skills on another person! Chest compressions can be dangerous to a conscious, healthy person but lifesaving for the cardiac arrest victim.

---

*Thanks to Allan Braslow, PhD, for coining the term *pump and blow* to describe chest compressions and rescue breathing.

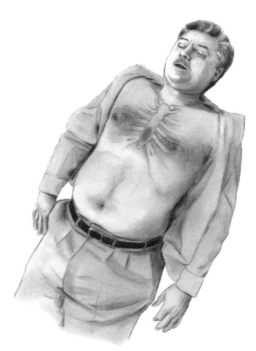

FIGURE 7.
Position for chest compressions, on the lower half of the sternum.

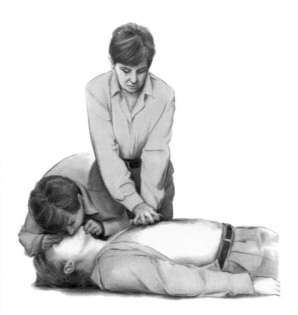

FIGURE 8.
Rescue breathing and compressions.

CRITICAL CONCEPTS: THE RECOVERY POSITION
HOW TO PLACE A PERSON IN THE RECOVERY POSITION IF UNCONSCIOUS BUT BREATHING

If there is no evidence of trauma, place the victim on his or her side in the *recovery position* (FIGURE 9). The recovery position keeps the airway open. The following steps are recommended:

1. Kneel beside the victim and straighten the victim's legs.

2. Place the victim's arm that is nearest you in a "waving good-bye" position, that is, at right angles to the victim's body, elbow bent, palm up.

3. Place the victim's other arm across his or her chest, as pictured below. If the victim is small, bring this arm further across so that the back of the hand can be held against the victim's nearest cheek.

4. Grasp the victim's far-side thigh above the knee; pull the thigh up toward the victim's body (FIGURE 9A).

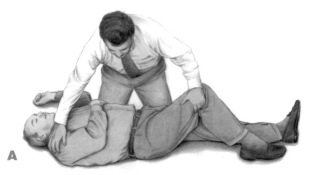

A

5. Place your other hand on the victim's far-side shoulder, and roll the victim toward you onto his or her side (FIGURE 9B). Begin moving the victim's uppermost hand toward the victim's nearest cheek (the hand must not get trapped under the body).

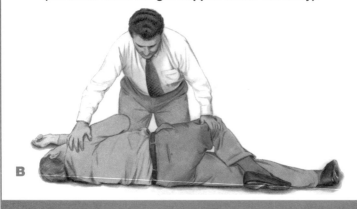

B

6. Adjust the upper leg of the knee you are holding until both the hip and knee are bent at right angles.

7. Tilt the victim's head back to keep the airway open. Bring the back of the uppermost hand under the victim's cheek. Use this hand to maintain head tilt. Use chin lift if necessary.

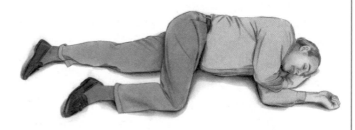

FIGURE 9.
The recovery position.

Continue to check the victim:

8. Check breathing regularly ("look, listen, and feel").

9. If the victim stops breathing, turn the victim onto his or her back, be sure that 911 has been called and the AED is near, and begin the ABCs of CPR.

10. *Memory aid: Victim is waving good-bye while taking a nap.*

BARRIER DEVICES AND MASKS

When you perform CPR, you have almost no chance of becoming infected with viral diseases such as AIDS or hepatitis. To date no human has ever "caught" AIDS or hepatitis by mouth-to-mouth contact during CPR.

Many rescuers, however, prefer to avoid direct mouth-to-mouth contact with another person, especially a stranger. The AHA recommends that you learn to use a barrier device to avoid direct mouth-to-mouth contact with a victim. But a barrier device is *not* required to provide CPR. **Do not withhold rescue breathing from a cardiac arrest victim just because you have no barrier device.**

There are 2 types of barrier devices: face shields and face masks.

Face Shields

Face shields are clear plastic or silicon sheets placed over the victim's face to keep the rescuer's mouth from directly touching the victim. All face shields have an opening or tube in the center of the plastic sheet. This allows your rescue breaths to enter the victim's mouth. Face shields are small, flexible, and portable. A shield will fit easily on a key ring. If you keep it on your key ring, it is much more likely to be available when you need it.

Face Masks

Face masks **(FIGURE 10)** are firmer, more rigid devices that fit over both the mouth and nose. Masks are much more effective than face shields, but they are bulkier, they cost more, and they're less likely to be available. Face masks and disposable gloves should be packed in every AED carrying case.

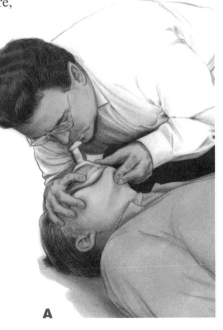
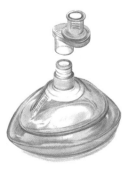

FIGURE 10.
Face mask.

A

CRITICAL CONCEPTS: THE VALUE OF CPR

Perform CPR to maintain circulation while getting the AED. Give CPR at all times *except* when attaching the electrode pads to the chest, analyzing, charging, and shocking VF. Remember, defibrillation is the only treatment that can convert VF to a normal heart rhythm. CPR is a temporary procedure to provide oxygen-rich blood to the brain and heart until the victim is successfully defibrillated.

TWO-RESCUER CPR

CPR can also be performed by two rescuers. One rescuer assesses the victim and provides rescue breathing. The second rescuer gives chest compressions. With two rescuers you change the ratio of chest compressions and rescue breaths from 15 pumps and 2 blows to 5 pumps and 1 blow each cycle.

Two-rescuer CPR is not covered in the standard Heartsaver AED Course. However, your course director may add two-person CPR. The instructor will provide a two-rescuer CPR performance sheet if needed in your course.

FOUNDATION FACTS: CHOOSING A FACE MASK

Face masks should

- Be easy to apply to the face
- Provide a good seal between mask and face
- Have a one-way valve with a bacterial barrier to keep the victim's exhaled air and body fluids away from the rescuer's mouth
- Be transparent so that the rescuer can see vomit or foreign material in the victim's airway

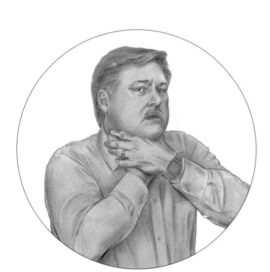

FIGURE 11.
Universal sign of choking distress.

In the Heartsaver AED Course you will learn about the specific face mask you will use during rescue breathing and CPR. Correct use requires practice. Practice on a manikin several times. The most critical step in using a face mask is achieving a good seal around the mouth and nose because this prevents air leakage during rescue breaths (FIGURE 10A).

CHOKING: AIRWAY OBSTRUCTION BY A FOREIGN BODY

Choking is an alarming and dramatic emergency. The desperate efforts of the choking person to clear his or her airway heighten the emotional drama and increase the pressure on the rescuer to take the correct action.

FOUNDATION FACTS: CAUSES OF AIRWAY OBSTRUCTION

There are 3 common ways an adult's airway may become obstructed. Each is treated differently.

1. **Foreign body.** A foreign body (for example, food) may become lodged in the air passage and block the airway. If the victim is an adult, give abdominal thrusts (Heimlich maneuver) or chest thrusts and finger sweeps (discussed below).

2. **Relaxed tongue.** In an unconscious victim (for example, after a stroke or head trauma or in cardiac arrest), the tongue may fall back against the throat, blocking the airway. Use either the head tilt–chin lift maneuver or the jaw-thrust maneuver to lift the tongue away from the back of the throat. (SEE FIGURES 3 AND 6.)

3. **Swollen air passages.** This condition is a medical problem rather than a mechanical problem. Swelling and blockage of the airway are caused by conditions such as asthma, infection, or allergy. Positioning of the head or neck and using the Heimlich maneuver will not eliminate this form of airway obstruction. If the victim stops breathing, give rescue breaths. Critical narrowing of the airway is a life-threatening condition. This condition cannot be resolved without using medications, such as epinephrine, or surgery.

How to Recognize Severe Airway Obstruction by a Foreign Body in a Conscious Victim

Foreign bodies may *partially* block the airway but still allow good air movement. These choking victims remain conscious, can cough forcefully, and usually can speak. Breath sounds may be noisy. These victims require no immediate action from you, but prepare to act if the airway obstruction worsens.

Victims with *severe* airway obstruction will remain conscious at first but will not be able to move enough air to cough forcefully. You must be prepared to help relieve the obstruction with abdominal thrusts.

To determine if a conscious victim has an obstructed airway, ask, "Are you choking?" In a conscious, choking person the following are *red flags* or major warning signs of severe airway obstruction that require you to act:

- *"Universal distress signal"* of choking: the victim clutches his or her neck with the thumb and index finger (FIGURE 11)
- Inability to speak (ask, "Are you choking?")
- Poor, ineffective coughs
- High-pitched sounds while inhaling
- Increased difficulty breathing
- Bluish skin color (cyanosis)
- Loss of consciousness if not treated immediately

NOTE ABOUT THE UNIVERSAL DISTRESS SIGNAL: You do not need to act if the victim can cough forcefully and speak. **Do not interfere** at this point because a strong cough is the most effective way to remove a foreign body. Stay with the victim and monitor his or her condition. If the partial obstruction persists, activate the EMS system.

First Aid for Airway Obstruction by a Foreign Body

Use the Heimlich maneuver (abdominal thrusts) to relieve severe airway obstruction caused by a foreign body. The Heimlich maneuver quickly forces air from the victim's lungs. This expels the blocking object like a cork from a bottle. Two approaches are used:

1. Use the **Heimlich maneuver** if the victim is *conscious* (but not speaking) and *standing* (FIGURE 12).

2. Use CPR skills **A (open the airway)** and **B (give rescue breaths)** plus **abdominal or chest thrusts (straddle the victim)** and **finger sweeps** if the victim is *unconscious* (FIGURE 13).

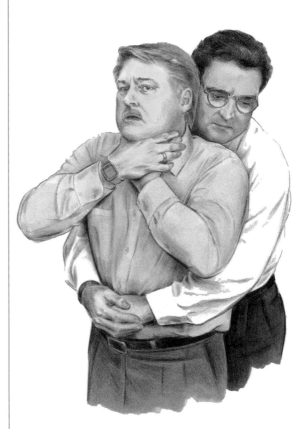

FIGURE 12.
Conscious-choking maneuver.

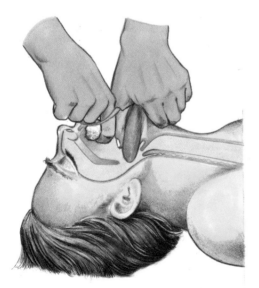

Figure 13.
Unconscious-choking maneuver: abdominal thrusts.

Figure 14.
Unconscious-choking maneuver: finger sweep.

If the choking victim is *conscious* and *standing:* perform the Heimlich maneuver:

1. Make a fist with one hand.

2. Place the thumb side of the fist on the victim's abdomen, slightly above the navel and well below the breastbone.

3. Grasp the fist with the other hand and provide quick upward thrusts into the victim's abdomen.

4. Repeat the thrusts and continue until the object is expelled or the victim becomes unconscious.

If the foreign-body airway obstruction is not relieved, the victim will stop breathing. Then the brain and heart will lack oxygen-rich blood. The victim will lose consciousness and become unresponsive. When the victim loses consciousness, ***activate the EMS system by calling 911 and get the AED.*** Then perform the *unconscious-choking maneuver* described below.

If the choking victim becomes *unconscious:* perform finger sweep, straddle the victim, use the Heimlich maneuver:

1. Place the victim on his or her back.

2. Grasp the tongue and jaw with one hand. Perform a finger sweep with the index finger of the other hand (**Figure 14**).

3. Attempt rescue breathing.

4. If the chest does not rise, reposition the victim's head and try blowing again.

5. If the victim's chest still does not rise with your breaths, perform the Heimlich maneuver for an unconscious victim:

   • Straddle the victim.

   • Place the heel of one hand on the abdomen just above the navel and well below the breastbone.

   • Place the heel of the other hand on top of the first.

   • Give up to 5 quick abdominal thrusts.

6. Repeat finger sweeps, rescue breaths, and abdominal thrusts until the obstruction is cleared.

First Aid for Choking in Pregnant and Obese Victims:
Conscious and Unconscious

When choking victims are in the later stages of pregnancy or are very obese, you must position your hands on the chest rather than on the abdomen to deliver thrusts.

Obese or Pregnant Choking Victim — Conscious:

1. Stand behind the victim and put your arms around the victim's chest.
2. Place your fist on the middle of the victim's breastbone between the nipples (take care to avoid the lower tip of the breastbone).
3. Grab your fist with your other hand and perform firm backward thrusts.
4. Repeat thrusts until the object is removed or the victim becomes unconscious.

Obese or Pregnant Choking Victim — Unconscious:

1. Place the victim on his or her back.
2. Grasp the victim's tongue and jaw with one hand. Perform a finger sweep with the index finger of the other hand **(FIGURE 14)**.
3. Try to give rescue breaths.
4. If the victim's chest does not rise: reposition the victim's head and try again.
5. If the victim's chest still does not rise with your breaths, perform chest thrusts:
   - *Do not* straddle the victim. Work from the side.
   - Place the heel of one hand on top of the other. Then place the heel of the lower hand on the center of the breastbone at the nipple line (similar to chest compressions of CPR).
   - Position your body directly over your hands (similar to chest compressions of CPR).
   - Give up to 5 firm chest thrusts.
6. Repeat finger sweeps, breathing attempts, and chest thrusts until the obstruction is cleared.

SUMMARY

The ABCs of CPR are an important first aid skill that everyone should know. In your lifetime you will probably encounter at least one emergency in which your ability to perform the ABCs will help save someone's life or prevent an urgent problem from becoming a life-threatening emergency.

Problems with **A**irway are common. Everyone should know the steps to take for

- Opening the airway of an unconscious victim
- Rescuing a choking victim who is distressed but still conscious
- Rescuing a choking victim who becomes unconscious
- First aid for choking in pregnant or obese victims, both conscious and unconscious

Problems with **B**reathing occur in these emergencies:

- Respiratory and cardiac arrest
- Stroke and seizure victims
- Victims of head trauma
- Drowning and near-drowning victims
- Victims of medication overdoses and drug intoxication

To manage **B**reathing problems, you need to know how to open the airway and give rescue breaths.

Finally, *chest compressions* (for **C**irculation) are needed in emergencies in which the victim also has no pulse. The most common cause of loss of a pulse is sudden cardiac arrest due to VF. The actions of pumping are simple and easy to learn.

The next chapter covers the use of AEDs, a seemingly technical skill that is easier to learn, as a matter of fact, than the skills of CPR.

REVIEW QUESTIONS

1. You are helping someone who is unresponsive. Which of the following groups of actions includes major steps of CPR in the correct order?

   a. call 911, check for a pulse, open the airway, give 2 breaths if needed

   b. open the airway, give 2 breaths if needed, check for a pulse, call 911 if no pulse

   c. call 911, open the airway, give 2 breaths if needed, and check for a pulse

   d. give 2 breaths, check for a pulse, call 911, begin chest compressions

2. You hear a colleague cry out in the next room. You enter the room and find a man collapsed on the floor. Your first step in assessing the situation is to

   a. check for breathing

   b. check the pulse

   c. check for responsiveness

   d. open the airway

3. If the victim is unresponsive, you perform a head tilt–chin lift and look, listen, and feel for breathing. If the victim is not breathing, what should you do next?

   a. give 2 rapid breaths

   b. give 2 slow breaths

   c. give 1 slow breath

   d. give 1 rapid breath

   e. begin chest compressions

4. For step **C** of the **ABCs,** where should you feel for the pulse of an unconscious adult victim?

   a. the wrist

   b. the neck

   c. the thigh

   d. the upper arm

5. What is the correct ratio of compressions (pumping) to ventilations (blowing) when performing one-rescuer CPR on an adult victim?

   a. 15 compressions to 2 ventilations

   b. 10 compressions to 2 ventilations

   c. 5 compressions to 2 ventilations

   d. 5 compressions to 1 ventilation

6. Which of the following is the most critical step when using a mouth-to-mask device?

    a. achieving a good seal around the mouth and nose

    b. using a two-way valve

    c. using a nontransparent mask

    d. blowing rapidly with each breath

7. What is the best way to ensure a proper rescue breath?

    a. see a change in the victim's color

    b. check the victim's pulse regularly

    c. see the victim's chest rise during rescue breathing

    d. check the airway frequently

8. You try to give a rescue breath to a victim and find that you cannot blow in easily and the victim's chest does not rise. What should you do immediately?

    a. use the Heimlich maneuver

    b. do a finger sweep

    c. reposition the head and try a rescue breath again

    d. give a more forceful breath

9. A conscious adult victim is clutching his throat and cannot speak, breathe, or cough. What should you do immediately?

    a. give abdominal thrusts

    b. give several back blows

    c. call 911

    d. check the airway

HOW DID YOU DO?
1. c; 2. c; 3. b; 4. b; 5. a; 6. a; 7. c; 8. c; 9. a

CONTENTS

3

LEARNING OBJECTIVES

1. Describe the purpose of an AED.

2. List the 4 universal steps required to operate all AEDs.

3. Describe the details of the 4 universal steps.

4. Describe the proper procedure for attaching the AED electrode pads in the correct positions on the victim's chest.

5. Explain why no one should touch the victim while the AED is analyzing, charging, or shocking the victim.

6. List at least 3 special conditions that might change your actions when using an AED.

7. Describe the proper actions to take when the AED indicates *"no shock indicated"* (or *"no shock advised"*).

8. Discuss how to maintain an AED.

WHAT IS AN AUTOMATED EXTERNAL DEFIBRILLATOR?

An *automated external defibrillator* (AED) is a computerized defibrillator (**FIGURE 1**). An AED can

- Analyze the heart rhythm of a person in cardiac arrest
- Recognize a shockable rhythm
- Advise the operator (through voice prompts and lighted indicators) whether the rhythm should be shocked

If a shock is indicated, the AED charges to a preset energy level. When the operator presses a SHOCK button, the AED delivers a shock to the cardiac arrest victim.

AEDs are relatively inexpensive and need little maintenance. They can be operated easily with very little training. Because of their effectiveness and ease of use and care, they are now being placed on airplanes and in public buildings, homes, and worksites. With more rescuers and more AEDs available, defibrillation can occur within minutes of a cardiac arrest.

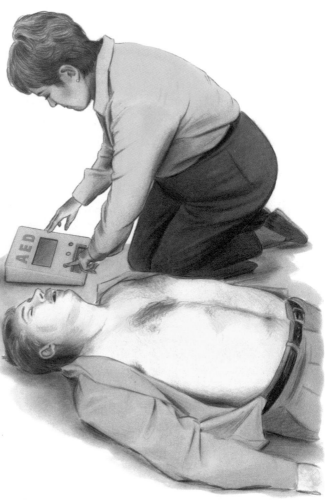

FIGURE 1.
An automated external defibrillator.

How an AED Analyzes the Heart Rhythm

AEDs contain computer chips that analyze the rate, size, and wave shape of the human cardiac rhythm. AEDs have been tested and are very accurate for use with adults.

AED electrode pads have 2 functions:

- To sense the cardiac electric signal and send it to the computer
- To deliver a shock through the electrodes if a shock is indicated

AEDs look at the victim's heart to see if it has a rhythm that can be shocked. If it does, the AED will tell you that a shock is advised. All AEDs must charge before they can deliver a shock. Some AEDs charge automatically. With some AEDs you have to press a CHARGE button before they will charge. You can then push another button to deliver the shock.

Overview: The 4 Universal Steps for Operating an AED

Like automobiles, AEDs are available in different models. There are small differences from model to model, but (like cars) all AEDs operate basically the same way. Do not be distracted by minor differences. Focus instead on the 4 universal steps you must perform with all AEDs. They are listed in the sidebar.

Special Conditions That May Require Additional Actions

When you arrive with an AED at the scene of a possible cardiac arrest, or if you are doing CPR and someone else arrives with an AED, quickly look for "special conditions" that may change how you use the AED. These are listed in the box on the next page.

Place the AED Next to the Victim's Left Ear

Make sure you have enough room to perform CPR and operate the AED. Do not attempt CPR in a bed, for example, or with the victim slumped over in a car or a chair. Place the victim on a firm surface, such as the floor. If possible, place the AED next to the victim's left ear. This allows you to easily reach the AED controls, place the adhesive electrode pads in the proper location, and direct CPR. However, this may not always be possible because of the circumstances and location of the collapse.

**CRITICAL CONCEPTS:
4 UNIVERSAL STEPS
OF AED OPERATION**

1. POWER ON the AED first!
2. ATTACH the AED to the patient's chest with electrode pads.
3. ANALYZE the rhythm.
4. SHOCK (if a shock is indicated).

CRITICAL CONCEPTS: SPECIAL SITUATIONS IN AED USE

1. *Water: Is the victim lying in water (for example, the wet surfaces around a swimming pool)?* Shocking on a wet surface may cause burns or shocks to the victim or rescuers.

   Actions:

   - Remove the victim from contact with water.
   - Drag the victim gently by the arms or legs, or use a blanket drag.
   - Dry the victim's chest quickly before attaching the AED.

2. *Metal surface: Is the victim lying on a metal surface?* Avoid shocking a victim who is lying on a metal surface. Because all metal conducts electric current, there is a small but unlikely risk of the electric charge shocking a rescuer or bystander near the patient.

   Action:

   - Remove the victim from contact with a metal surface.

3. *Children: Is the victim a child younger than 8 years?* AEDs have been tested and approved by the FDA only for children 8 years old (or older). In addition, the electric energy settings of AEDs are often too high for children under 8 years old.

   Action:

   - If the victim is younger than 8 years, do not use the AED.

4. *Transdermal medications: Do patch medications interfere with placement of electrode pads on the victim's chest?* Placing an AED electrode pad on top of a medication patch may block delivery of shocks or cause small burns to the skin.

   Action:

   - Remove the patch and wipe the area clean before attaching the AED.

5. *Implanted pacemakers or defibrillators: Does the victim have a pacemaker or implanted cardioverter-defibrillator?* These devices create a hard lump beneath the skin of the upper chest or abdomen (usually on the victim's left side). The lump is about half the size of a deck of cards and usually has a small overlying scar. Placing an AED electrode pad directly over an implanted medical device may reduce the effectiveness of defibrillation.

   Actions:

   - Do not place an AED electrode pad directly over an implanted device.
   - Place an AED electrode pad at least 1 inch to the side of any implanted device.

FOLLOWING THE UNIVERSAL STEPS OF AED OPERATION

In chapter 4 we will "put it all together" and blend your CPR skills with AED operation. This section covers specific details you should know about using an AED in a real situation. These details are summarized in the box on the left. Remember, these steps start only *after* you have verified that the victim is unresponsive, is not breathing, and has no pulse and you have placed the AED near the victim's left ear. You will practice and rehearse real-life situations during the Heartsaver AED practice scenario sessions.

Step 1. POWER ON the AED first! (FIGURE 2)

a. ***Open the AED.*** This automatically turns the *power on* in some devices.

b. ***Press the POWER ON button first.***
This is critical because sound alerts, lights, and voice prompts will tell you that the power is ON and will direct you through the steps of using the AED. Always turn the AED ON as the first step. Do *not* wait until you have opened the package of adhesive electrode pads or attached the electrode pads to the patient's chest.

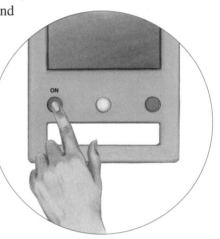

FIGURE 2.
Operate AED; POWER ON first.

Step 2. ATTACH adhesive electrode pads to the victim's chest (stop CPR chest compressions) (FIGURE 3).

a. ***Remove clothing from the victim's chest.*** Place 2 adhesive electrode pads directly on the skin of the victim's chest. The chest should be bare to the skin. Remove clothing and undergarments as needed, even for women. Do not hesitate — remember that you are trying to save the victim's life. Bandage scissors can be stored in the AED carrying case to cut clothing that is hard to remove.

b. ***Dry the victim's chest if necessary.*** *Be sure* the victim's chest is bare and wiped dry. This will help the AED electrode pads stick firmly so that they will not shift or fall off during defibrillation. Keep a cloth or gauze in the AED carrying case for drying.

c. ***Open the package of adhesive electrode pads in the AED carrying case.*** Some defibrillation electrode pads are preconnected to the cables. For others, join one end of the cable to the AED. Then attach the other end of the cable to the electrode pads.

d. ***Join ("snap") the connecting cables to the electrode pads (in some AEDs the cables are preconnected to the electrode pads).*** First put the electrode pads on the floor or the ground. Then snap the cables down on the pad connecting posts *before* you place the pads on the patient's chest.

e. ***Attach the adhesive electrode pads to the victim's chest (stop CPR chest compressions during this step to ensure proper pad placement).*** Peel away the protective plastic backing from the electrode pads to expose the adhesive surface. Attach the AED electrode pads, adhesive side down, directly to the skin of the victim's chest. Follow the example pictured on the pad packaging. It is not necessary to match position and cable alignment exactly, but try to place the pads like those in the example.

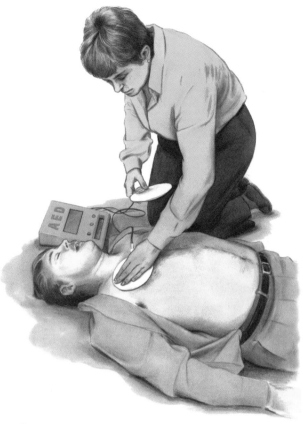

FIGURE 3.
Attach AED.

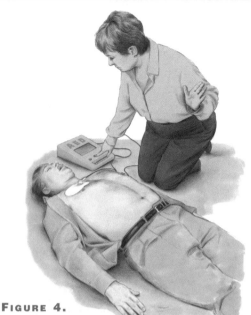

FIGURE 4.
"Clear" during analysis.

FOUNDATION FACTS: MAKING THE CONNECTIONS

AEDs require that 4 objects be connected in a line: from the AED, to the connecting cable, to the AED electrode pads, to the patient's chest. Remember

1. The **AED** is joined to the

2. **Connecting cables,** which are joined to the

3. **AED electrode pads,** which are attached to

4. The **victim's chest**

AED manufacturers have not yet standardized these connections. Learn these details of your particular AED during the course. In newer AED models the electrode pads are preattached to the connecting cables, and the connecting cables are preattached to the AED. All the operator has to do is open the electrode pad package and attach the pads to the patient's chest.

Learn exactly how much of the AED "circuit" you must put together for your AED *before* you need it in an emergency. Remember that you can figure out the connections by recalling the 4 elements that must be joined: *AED, cables, electrode pads, patient* (FIGURE 5).

---

f. **Proper pad locations.** The *first pad* goes on the *upper right side* of the victim's chest, to the right of the breastbone, between the nipple and collarbone. The second pad goes to the outside of the left nipple, with the top margin of the pad several inches below the left armpit. Follow the example on the package. The AED will operate even if pad placement is not exactly as pictured.

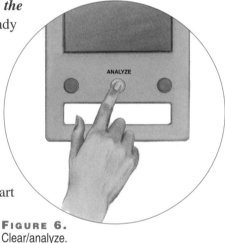

FIGURE 5.
Chest-to-AED circuit.

Step 3. ANALYZE the victim's rhythm (FIGURES 4, 5, 6).

a. **Stop CPR. Do not touch the victim.** When you are ready to analyze the victim's rhythm, stop CPR completely. *Do not touch the victim or have any physical contact with the victim* (FIGURE 4) (because it could interfere with AED analysis). Some AEDs start to analyze the rhythm as soon as the electrode pads are attached. Others require you to push an ANALYZE button to start rhythm analysis. From this point forward — whenever the machine is analyzing, preparing to shock, or actually delivering the shock to the victim — it is critical that you, your team members, and all bystanders avoid *all* contact with the victim.

FIGURE 6.
Clear/analyze.

b. **Announce, "Stand clear of the patient!"** The rescuer operating the AED should state clearly, *"Stand clear of the patient! Analyzing rhythm! Stand clear!"* You do not need to use these exact words, but make sure the message gets across. *No one should touch the victim during analysis or shock.* If anyone is touching the victim, refuse to push the ANALYZE or SHOCK buttons until contact with the victim stops.

Step 4. Charge the AED and deliver the SHOCK (if indicated) (**FIGURE 7**).

a. ***Stay clear while charging.*** When the AED recognizes a shockable rhythm, voice messages will prompt you to "stay clear." Most AED models begin charging automatically. You must make sure that no one is touching the victim. To prepare for shock delivery, announce and verify (with a visual check), *"I'm clear, you're clear, we're all clear."*

b. ***Push to shock.*** When charging is complete, the machine will advise you to *"push to shock."* Just before you press the SHOCK button, *make one last check to be sure that no one is touching the victim.* Then press the SHOCK button to deliver the shock to the victim.

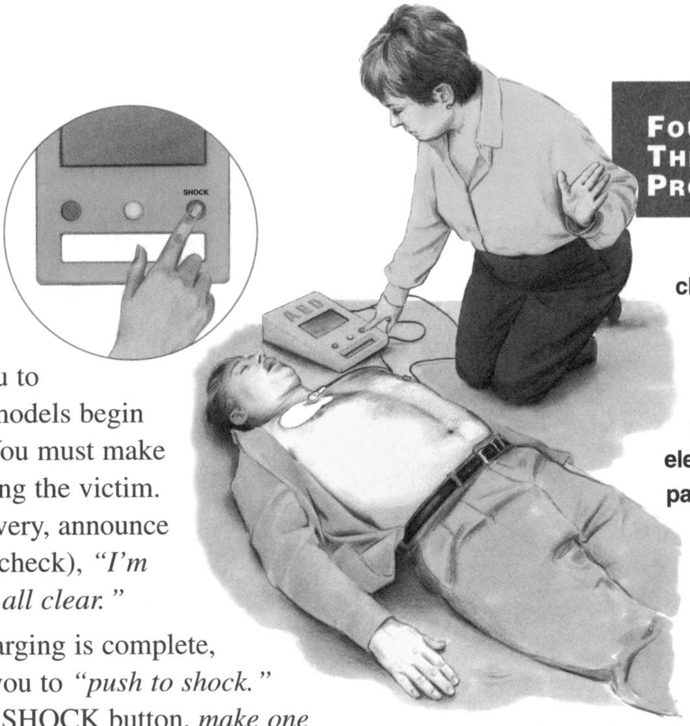

c. ***Follow the shock sequence:***
   - *Analyze, shock*
   - *Analyze, shock*
   - *Analyze, shock*

The number of shocks an AED delivers and the energy level for each shock are preset by the manufacturer. Let the AED follow the shock sequence it has been programmed to deliver. Follow the AED voice and visual prompts. Continue to follow the sequence of actions outlined in chapter 4 until EMS personnel arrive. Transfer the care of the victim to EMS personnel after the AED has completed the shock cycles.

If **"no shock indicated,"** *check pulse. Then begin sequence of CPR.*

a. ***Leave AED electrode pads attached. Check ABCs.*** If the victim's heart is no longer in VF, the AED will signal *"no shock indicated"* (or *"no shock advised"*) or *"check breathing and pulse."* Leave the AED electrodes attached to the victim's chest. Check for a pulse. Then follow the ABCs of CPR.

FIGURE 7.
Shock.

If the victim has a hairy chest, the adhesive electrode pads may stick to the hair of the chest so that contact is not made with the skin on the chest. This will lead to a "check electrodes" or "check electrode pads" message on the AED. Try the following:

- Press down firmly on each pad. That may solve the problem.

- Quickly pull off the electrode pads. This will remove much of the chest hair. Dry the chest and apply a second set of electrode pads. See if the AED will now analyze.

- If you still cannot get a good connection, pull off the second set of electrode pads. Then shave the area for pad placement with a few strokes of the prep razor in the AED carrying case. Then open and apply a new (third) set of electrode pads.

Professional responders are given plastic disposable razors to quickly shave a suitable area of chest hair so that the electrode pads stick directly to the skin. Consider whether you are comfortable with the idea of shaving someone's chest after practicing the Heartsaver AED scenarios. Two of these razors should be packed in the AED storage case with 2 extra sets of electrode pads.

CRITICAL CONCEPTS: PAD PLACEMENT

Practice opening the electrode pad package and attaching the cables while your partner performs CPR, including rescue breathing and chest compressions. When you are ready to apply the electrode pads, remove the adhesive backing of the first pad. Then stop CPR chest compressions. Quickly apply the pads and allow the AED to analyze the rhythm. With some AEDs you may have to press the ANALYZE button. Other AEDs will automatically analyze as soon as the electrode pads are properly attached.

You may receive a voice prompt or alarm if the electrode pads are not securely attached to the chest or if the cables are not fastened properly. The voice warning will state *"check pads"* or *"check electrodes,"* or words to that effect. Troubleshoot by checking the following:

1. If the victim has a hairy chest, try removing and reapplying the pads or shaving the chest (see "The Hairy Chest Problem").

2. Are the electrode pads stuck firmly and evenly to the skin of the chest?

3. Are the cables correctly connected to the adhesive electrode pads?

4. Are the cables correctly connected to the AED?

When you correct the problem, most AEDs will automatically go into the analyze mode.

b. *If the victim is breathing adequately and has a pulse,* place the victim in the **recovery position** and monitor breathing until EMS personnel arrive.

c. *If the victim is not breathing but has a pulse,* give rescue breaths (1 breath every 5 seconds). Check the pulse frequently **(FIGURE 8).**

d. *If the victim is not breathing and has no pulse,* resume CPR.

e. *Care after shock.* Leave the AED electrode pads in place and the AED turned ON. *Do **NOT** remove the electrode pads or turn the*

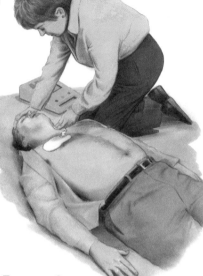

FIGURE 8.
Pulse check.

CRITICAL CONCEPTS: AED MAINTENANCE

- Become familiar with your AED and how it operates.
- Check the AED for any visible problems, such as open case or sign of damage.
- Check the "ready-for-use" indicator on your AED (if so equipped) daily.
- Perform any other user-based maintenance according to the manufacturer's recommendation.
- Check to see that the AED carrying case contains the following minimum accessories:
  - 2 sets of *spare* defibrillator electrode pads (3 total)
  - 2 pocket face masks
  - 1 extra battery (if appropriate for your AED; some AEDs have batteries that last for years)
  - 2 prep razors (supplied by manufacturers)
  - 5 to 10 alcohol wipes
  - 5 sterile gauze pads (4 × 4 inches), individually wrapped
  - 1 absorbent cloth towel

Remember: AED malfunctions are extremely rare. Most reported problems have been caused by failure to perform user-based maintenance of the AED.

AED off until instructed to do so by EMS personnel. The victim may "rearrest" and lose spontaneous respirations and pulse. If the AED is always ready for use, you and others on your rescue team can resume the AED action sequence as soon as it is needed.

AED MAINTENANCE AND TROUBLESHOOTING

Newer models of AEDs require almost no maintenance. They can check themselves to see if they are working and ready for use. But you and your coworkers who are trained to use an AED must still make sure your AED is ready for use at a moment's notice.

AED manufacturers provide specific recommendations about checking maintenance and readiness. See the handout *Manufacturer's Instructions and Guide to Maintenance* that your instructor will have. Your instructor will give you information about the type of maintenance your AED needs or refer you to a source of more information.

SUMMARY

Do not become confused by the details presented in this chapter. AEDs are simple, easy to use, and user friendly. Many people who take a Heartsaver AED course need only a few minutes to get the "big picture" of operating an AED and then spend time practicing:

- POWER ON the AED first. Listen to the voice and visual prompts.
- ATTACH the electrode pads (paying attention to the figures on pad location and stopping chest compressions).
- ANALYZE the rhythm (this may occur automatically).
- Press the SHOCK button if shock is indicated (clear the patient first).

These are the only defibrillation steps most lay rescuers using an AED will ever need to know. Performing these same steps during an actual VF arrest will get the job done.

Other lay responders, however, will appreciate the details about defibrillation presented in this chapter. If you are curious about the rich variety of "what if?" situations that can arise during defibrillation, this chapter will help answer your questions. It will also enrich your understanding of defibrillation.

CRITICAL CONCEPTS: NO ONE SHOULD TOUCH THE VICTIM

No one should touch the victim during
- **Analysis**
- **Charging**
- **Shocks**

If you touch or move the victim during the analyze mode, the AED might read the victim's cardiac rhythm incorrectly. Anyone touching the victim during shock delivery may receive a small shock. Although serious injury is very unlikely, there can be some pain and discomfort.

FOUNDATION FACTS: "IF'S"

Here are some challenging "if" statements that may seem confusing. Do not worry about each of the "if" possibilities. You and your instructor will practice them many times in class.

- **If the AED displays a *"shock indicated"* or *"shock advised"* message, press the SHOCK button.**
- **If the AED indicates *"no shock indicated,"* check for a pulse.**
- **If there is no pulse, resume compression-ventilation cycles (15:2) for 1 minute. Then check the pulse again.**
- **If no pulse is found, analyze the victim's rhythm again.**
- **After 3 *"no shock indicated"* messages, give 1 to 2 minutes of CPR.**
- **Repeat the analyze period every 1 to 2 minutes as you continue to do CPR.**

REVIEW QUESTIONS

1. What is an AED?

   a. a heart monitor that tells you when to start CPR

   b. a device used to treat victims of cardiac arrest who fail to respond to 15 minutes of CPR

   c. a device to analyze the adult heart for a shockable rhythm and to deliver defibrillation shocks

   d. a device that electrically "paces" the heart at 60 to 80 beats per minute

2. In correct order, what are the 4 universal steps required to operate an AED?

   a. POWER ON, ATTACH the electrode pads to the victim's chest and to the AED, ANALYZE the victim's rhythm, and deliver a SHOCK if needed

   b. call 911, begin CPR, use the AED, and provide advanced life support

   c. move the victim to a safe place, attach the electrode pads to the victim's chest, attach the cables to the electrode pads, and attach the cables to the AED

   d. check for a pulse, POWER ON, deliver a shock, and then analyze the victim's rhythm

HOW DID YOU DO?

1. c;   2. a

CONTENTS

4

LEARNING OBJECTIVES

After reading this section, you should be able to

1. List the criteria for when to start CPR and use the AED

2. Describe the 3 assessment steps for a collapsed person

3. Describe the roles for lay rescuers with an AED

4. Demonstrate how to manage the following collapsed victims with an AED when you are given a scenario:

   - No shock advised, no pulse

   - Shock advised, single shock, return of pulse and breathing

   - Shock advised, 3 shocks in a row, CPR for 1 minute, return of pulse after the fourth shock

5. Describe how you can help a victim of cardiac arrest even if no AED is available

INTRODUCTION

In this chapter you will learn to combine the skills of CPR (chapter 2) with your knowledge of using an AED (chapter 3). You will learn a simple algorithm (a set of steps) for most rescue situations you will encounter. The Heartsaver AED algorithm guides you whether you respond to a cardiac arrest as a single rescuer alone or with others who can help. The AEDs you will use will provide audio and visual prompts at every step, including CPR and defibrillation. You have only a few steps to memorize and a few decisions to make along the way. Your major learning task is to become familiar with the steps you will perform during the "pump and blow" of CPR and how to open, attach, and use the AED. The chapter ends with several practice scenarios to review what you have learned and to cover several possible outcomes of your rescue efforts.

MAINTAINING THE CHAIN OF SURVIVAL

Whether you respond to a cardiovascular emergency at home, at the worksite, or in the community, you can be the start of a strong Chain of Survival. The links in the Chain of Survival are early activation of the EMS system, early CPR, early defibrillation, and early advanced care. The call to 911 activates the EMS system and brings a professional emergency care team to the scene. The CPR you provide maintains the heart in a condition that favors successful defibrillation. When advanced EMS personnel arrive at the scene, they will help stabilize the patient and give additional treatments that increase the chance of successful resuscitation. This is especially true for victims who are not in ventricular fibrillation.

Defibrillation sounds complicated, but it is actually easier than CPR.

WHEN TO START CPR?
WHEN TO USE THE AED?

Here are 3 major cues for starting CPR and using the AED. You need to remember them. All 3 conditions must be present to start CPR and use the AED.

- *Unresponsiveness:* This prompts you to take 2 actions: call 911 *and* get the AED.

- *Not breathing:* This prompts you to give rescue breathing.

- *No pulse:* This prompts you to take 2 actions: use the AED and start chest compressions.

At this point you really don't have to make decisions. Just recognize the 3 conditions: **unresponsive, not breathing, no pulse.** Know the action you must take in response.

When the AED is turned on, attached to the patient, and placed in analyze mode, it will identify one of two conditions: *shockable rhythm present* or *shockable rhythm absent.* You respond to the AED prompts by "clearing" the patient, pressing the ANALYZE button (this is done automatically in some models), and pressing the SHOCK button when indicated. That's all there is to the use of the AED. Once you complete the use of the AED, you return to supporting the victim with CPR, rescue breathing, or the recovery position. EMS responders should arrive within a few short minutes.

ACTION SEQUENCE:
THE HEARTSAVER AED PROTOCOL

Combining CPR With Using an AED:
The Heartsaver AED Protocol

When you see a person who may be in cardiac arrest, act quickly but calmly. Follow the same sequences you learned for CPR (chapter 2) and AED operation (chapter 3). The Heartsaver AED Course teaches CPR and AED in 3 learning steps:

- *The steps of CPR*

- *The steps of AED operation*

- *The full action sequence of the Heartsaver AED protocol*

THE HEARTSAVER AED PROTOCOL

Unresponsive? 911 — AED

Check unresponsiveness: Shout, *"Are you OK?"*
If unresponsive:

Call 911! Point to another witness: *"You! Go call 911!"*
(Start CPR while witness goes for the AED. If alone, you must go yourself.)

AED: Get the AED located next to the telephone:
". . . And get the AED next to the phone!"
(If alone, you must get the AED yourself.)

(Return to the side of the victim.)

Start the ABCDs:

A: **A**irway open: head tilt–chin lift; jaw thrust.

B: **B**reathing check *(look, listen, and feel):*
if no breathing, give **2 slow breaths.**

C: **C**irculation check — **no pulse** is the signal to

- **Start chest compressions/begin rescue breathing**

plus

D: **D**efibrillation: **attach** and **operate** the AED

*(To continue, see next section,
"The 5-Step AED Treatment Protocol.")*

SUMMARY: THE HEARTSAVER AED PROTOCOL

A-B-C: The 4 Steps of CPR

1. Unresponsive?
   Call 911 — get the AED.
2. Airway: Perform head tilt–chin lift.
3. Breathing: *Look, listen, and feel.* Give 2 breaths if needed.
4. Circulation: Check pulse; start chest compressions if needed. (Stop during pad placement.)

D: The 4 Universal Steps of AED Operation

1. POWER ON the AED first!
2. ATTACH the AED to the victim's bare chest (AED, cables, pads).
3. ANALYZE rhythm.
4. SHOCK (if shock indicated).

The 5-Step AED Treatment Protocol

Attach and operate the AED:

1. POWER ON the AED first.

- Open carrying case or top of AED; turn AED **ON.**
  - *POWER ON allows voice and visual prompts from the AED to guide the operator.*
  - *POWER ON may occur automatically in some AEDs by opening the lid.*

2. ATTACH the AED to the patient.

- **Attach** AED connecting **cables** to the **AED.**
  - *May be preconnected in some AEDs.*
- **Attach** AED connecting **cables** to the adhesive chest electrode **pads.**
  - *May be preconnected.*
- **Attach** adhesive **pads** to patient's bare **chest** after peeling off backing.
  - *Stop chest compressions while placing AED electrode pads.*

3. ANALYZE the rhythm.

- **Clear** the patient before and during analysis; check that no one is touching the patient, including the person doing rescue breathing.
- **Press** the **ANALYZE** button to start rhythm analysis *(some brands of AEDs do not require this step).*

4. "Shock Sequence" (if indicated):

- **"Clear."** Clear patient once more before pushing the SHOCK button.
- **"SHOCK."** Press the SHOCK button to deliver the shock *(patient may display muscle contractions).*
- **"Clear."** *Clear the patient again before each analysis and shock.*
- **"ANALYZE."**
- **"Clear."** *Clear the patient again before each analysis and shock.*
- **"SHOCK."** Press the SHOCK button up to 2 more times if AED signals *"shock indicated."*

5. "No Shock Indicated" Sequence:

Check **pulse:**

- If **pulse:** check **breathing.**
  - If *inadequate* **breathing:** assist with rescue breathing (1 breath every 5 seconds).
  - If *adequate* **breathing:** place the victim in the recovery position.
- If no **pulse:** resume CPR for 1 minute; then **recheck** pulse.
- If no **pulse** after 1 minute, reanalyze rhythm: AED will indicate either *"shock indicated"* (go to step 4) or *"no shock indicated"* (repeat step 5).

Memorize the "shock indicated" *and* "no shock indicated" *sequences*

We highly recommend that you memorize 2 simple action sequences: *"shock indicated"* and *"no shock indicated."* The sequence you follow is based on the AED's rhythm analysis and the clinical responses of the victim. The AED will lead you through the 2 sequences. We will refer to these sequences throughout the Heartsaver AED handbook and course.

As long as the "shock indicated" message occurs, follow this sequence:

- Clear
- **SHOCK**
- Clear
- **ANALYZE**
- Repeat up to 3 shocks if needed; then resume CPR.

Whenever the "no shock indicated" message occurs, follow this sequence:

- Check **pulse.**
- If **pulse,** check **breathing.** *Inadequate:* assist breathing. *Adequate:* place the victim in the recovery position.
- If **no pulse,** resume CPR for 1 minute; then recheck pulse.
- If **no pulse,** analyze rhythm; then repeat the sequences: *"shock indicated"* or *"no shock indicated."*

Remember the 3 Conditions That Must Be Present to Start CPR or Use the AED

Recognize the 3 conditions and know the action you must take in response.

To start CPR or use the AED, victim must be

1. Unresponsive — call 911 *and* get the AED
2. Not breathing — give rescue breaths
3. Pulseless — use the AED *and* start compressions

Memorize the 2

action sequences:

"shock indicated"

and

"no shock indicated."

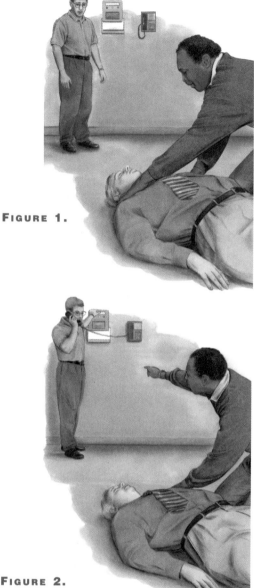

FIGURE 1.

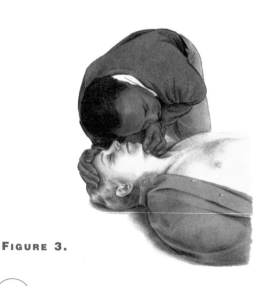

FIGURE 2.

APPLYING THE TWO-RESCUER HEARTSAVER AED ACTION SEQUENCE

Witnessed Arrest With Two People Responding

Chapters 2 and 3 show the one-rescuer scenario: a single person witnesses a collapse and must perform the entire Heartsaver AED action sequence. Another common scenario is the two-rescuer scenario: a witnessed arrest, such as at a worksite or a public place, with several bystanders. **FIGURES 1 THROUGH 14** demonstrate use of the Heartsaver AED action sequence for this scenario.

Two-Rescuer Heartsaver AED Action Sequence

- **Check unresponsiveness:** Shout, "Are you OK?" **(FIGURE 1)** If unresponsive:

- **Call 911!** Point to another witness: "You! Go call 911!"

- **AED:** Get the AED located next to the telephone: ". . . And get the AED next to the phone!" **(FIGURE 2)**

- The person who calls 911 gets the AED.

- The person who will use the AED stays with the victim.

  (These roles may be reversed in many circumstances.)

- The Heartsaver AED rescuer starts CPR during the call to 911.

- **A — Airway** open: head tilt–chin lift; jaw thrust **(FIGURE 3).**

  — If trauma is suspected, use the jaw-thrust maneuver to open the airway.

  — Face mask is available in AED carrying case.

  — Face shield is more likely to be available to first rescuer.

- **B — Breathing** check *(look, listen, and feel)* **(FIGURE 3).**

FIGURE 3.

- If no breathing, give 2 slow breaths **(FIGURE 4)**.

  — Key: Rescuer must see chest rise with each breath.

  — Face masks are the preferred barrier device, but face shields are acceptable.

  — Face masks should have a one-way valve.

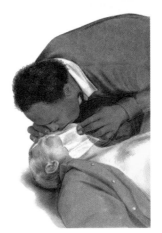

FIGURE 4.

- **C — Circulation:** check for a pulse **(FIGURE 5)**. Finding no pulse is the signal to

- Start chest compressions, begin rescue breathing, attach the AED.

  — Pulse checks are notoriously inaccurate; if there is any doubt, do chest compressions and use the AED.

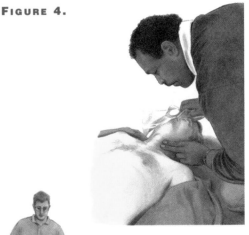

FIGURE 5.

- Remove clothing covering the chest. The victim's chest should be bare for chest compressions and using the AED.

- Use the landmark "center of chest, right between the nipples" to locate hand compression point **(FIGURE 6)**.

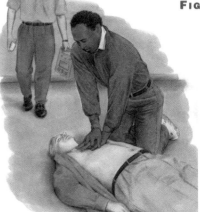

- The 911 caller delivers the AED to the person doing CPR.

- The 911 caller begins doing CPR **(FIGURE 7)**. (It is acceptable to reverse these roles.)

- The preferred AED placement is next to the victim's left ear, but this may not be possible in all cases.

FIGURE 6.

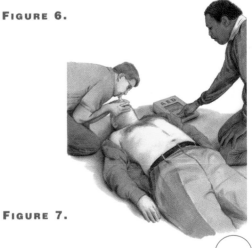

FIGURE 7.

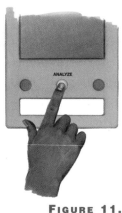

FIGURE 8.

- Open the carrying case or top of the AED.

- **POWER ON** the AED first **(FIGURE 8)** (some devices will turn on automatically when the AED lid or carrying case is opened).

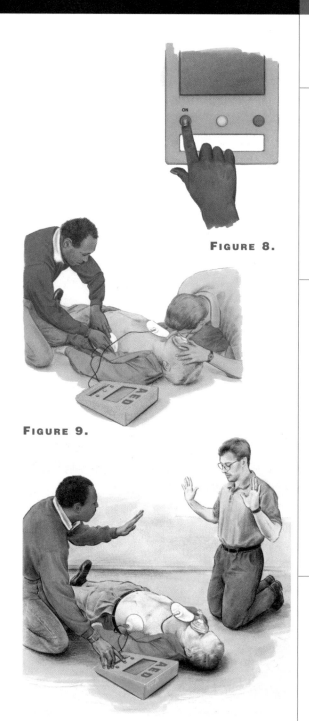

FIGURE 9.

- **ATTACH** AED connecting *cables* to the *AED* (may be preconnected).

- **ATTACH** AED connecting *cables* to the adhesive *electrode pads* (may be preconnected).

- **ATTACH** adhesive *electrode pads* to the patient's bare *chest* **(FIGURE 9).**

 — If necessary, stop chest compressions while placing AED electrode pads.

FIGURE 10.

- **ANALYZE** the rhythm.

- Clear the patient before and during analysis **(FIGURE 10).**

- Check that no one is touching the patient, including the person doing rescue breathing.

- Press the **ANALYZE** button to start rhythm analysis **(FIGURE 11)** (some brands of AEDs do not require this step).

FIGURE 11.

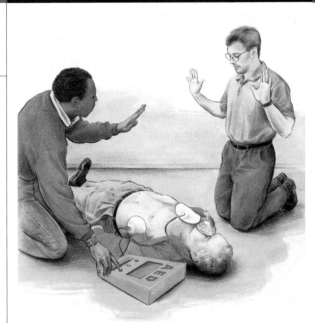

- *"Shock advised":* Follow the ***"shock indicated"*** sequence:

  — Clear the patient once more before pushing the SHOCK button **(FIGURE 12).**

  — Press the SHOCK button to deliver shock if the AED signals *"shock advised"* **(FIGURE 13)** (patient may display muscle contractions; continue to clear).

  — Press the ANALYZE and SHOCK buttons up to 2 more times if AED signals *"shock advised"* or *"shock indicated."* (Clear the patient again before each analysis and shock.)

FIGURE 12.

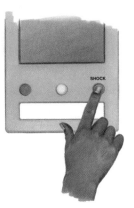

- Whenever the AED signals *"no shock indicated":* Follow the ***"no shock indicated"*** sequence:

  — Check the pulse **(FIGURE 14).**

  — If pulse, check breathing. If breathing is inadequate, assist breathing. If breathing is adequate, place the victim in the recovery position.

  — If no pulse, resume CPR for 1 minute; then recheck pulse.

  — If no pulse, analyze rhythm.

  — Then follow *"shock indicated"* or *"no shock indicated"* steps above.

FIGURE 13.

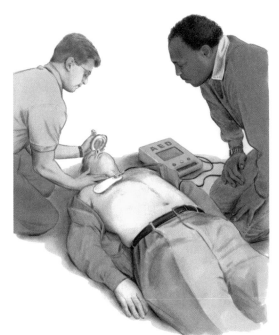

FIGURE 14.

. . . .

You must

make only

3 critical

assessments:

Unresponsive?

Breathing?

Pulse?

. . . .

THE HEARTSAVER RESCUER WITH AN AED: THE RESCUE DIRECTOR

In this course you will be trained to be the *rescue director*. You have the skills both to do CPR and operate an AED. In many rescue situations you may be the only witness who has either of these abilities. Although your responsibility is great, the tasks are simple — tell other witnesses to *"call 911 — get the AED located by the telephone";* tell other rescuers to *"help with CPR."* You will ensure that actions are taken in the proper sequence as quickly as possible and that they are well coordinated.

The bottom line — you must make only **3 critical assessments:** *unresponsive? breathing? pulse?* You learned these assessments in basic CPR. After that you simply follow prompts from the AED.

The beauty of AED technology is its simple design. Almost anyone can operate an AED. As you will see in the training video and demonstrations by your instructor, AEDs give you a lot of guidance: voice prompts, tone and light signals, and visual icons and figures on the device and defibrillator pads. Defibrillation sounds complicated, but you will see during practice sessions that operating an AED is easy. It is actually easier than learning and performing CPR.

As you mentally rehearse during this class and future practice sessions, think of yourself as the rescue director. When you think through several sample scenarios, you will realize that *You Can Do It!* Other witnesses will appreciate your knowledge, skills, and confidence. They will be happy to follow your directions and help where they can.

THE HEARTSAVER AED RESCUER WITH TWO OR MORE PEOPLE TO HELP

What happens when a cardiac arrest is witnessed by several people? They all want to help but may be unsure of what to do. In some worksites all employees will be trained as Heartsaver AED rescuers. Almost everyone will be knowledgeable and have a sense of what to do. The answer — *you direct them.* Unless you are alone, as a Heartsaver AED rescuer you should not leave the victim's side. If other witnesses are present, particularly other Heartsaver AED rescuers, *use them.* Direct them to perform one of these tasks:

- *Call 911.*
- *Get the AED.*
- *Do CPR: Do rescue breathing. Do chest compressions.*

You will practice these scenarios during the Heartsaver AED Course. The rescue tasks of calling 911, getting the AED, starting CPR, and operating the AED will be practiced in the 8 core scenarios, where the tasks will be divided several ways. In each scenario *the Heartsaver AED rescuer is the rescue director.* The Heartsaver AED rescuer will perform *both* the initial assessment and CPR and will operate the AED when it arrives.

Instructors may teach these roles another way: *whoever calls 911 and gets the AED will operate the AED*. This means that the second rescuer must be able to perform the initial ABCs and CPR. Either approach is acceptable. The preferred approach is for the AED rescuer to always remain with the victim.

A Heartsaver

AED rescuer

must know

how to

- *Give CPR*

- *Use an AED*

- *Put CPR and*

AED together.

You Can Do It!

THE HEARTSAVER AED RESCUER AND PROMPTS FROM THE AED

The AED is a remarkable electric device. One of its most useful features is the audio voice prompts that provide feedback to the Heartsaver AED rescuer. During the Heartsaver AED Course you will have many opportunities to practice and learn the audio and visual prompts of the specific AED you will use. All AED models provide at least 4 types of voice messages:

- *Analysis indicator:* when the AED is analyzing the rhythm *("analyzing; do not touch the patient").*

- *Shockable rhythm indicator:* whether or not the AED identifies a shockable rhythm during analysis *("shock indicated"* or *"no shock indicated").*

- *Loose electrode indicator:* *"check electrodes"* sounds when there is any break in the connections between the victim's skin and the AED. Most often this break occurs where the electrode pad contacts the skin, but the break can also occur at the cable-to-pad connections or at the cable-to-AED connections.

- *Sequencing information:* AEDs provide sequencing steps *("connect electrodes"* or *"check airway, check breathing, check pulse"* or *"perform CPR if no pulse").*

SUMMARY

This is the "putting-it-all-together" chapter. A trained Heartsaver AED rescuer must know how to give CPR, how to use an AED, and how to use the two together. Although most lay rescuers will respond with others to a witnessed cardiac arrest, many arrests occur in the home with only a distraught loved one to provide the first minutes of care. This chapter demonstrates how easy it is to integrate the two skills — CPR and AED — for use by a single, well-trained provider — the Heartsaver AED rescuer.

The cases below were carefully selected and developed to provide an overview of the major types of emergencies you are likely to encounter. Review the cases and try to answer the questions. This "thinking" exercise will strongly reinforce the ideas and skills you learn in the Heartsaver AED Course. In the course you will actually rehearse similar scenarios multiple times.

Study Cases

The following **study cases** let you review different situations that you may face as a Heartsaver AED rescuer. Do the following:

- Carefully review each case.
- Consider the single **best** answer to the case question.
- Write your answer in the space provided.
- In the answer section, review the correct answer and why it is the best answer.
- If the answer and discussion are unclear, review the related section in the handbook.
- If you have further questions, ask your Heartsaver AED Course instructor.

Case 1: Return of Pulse, Not Breathing

Your 50-year-old spouse clutches his or her chest while eating dinner and collapses on the floor. You verify unresponsiveness, call 911, and get the AED from near the telephone. You then assess the ABCs and find that your spouse is pulseless and not breathing. You attach the AED. You clear for analysis; the AED advises a shock. You deliver a shock, and the machine displays a no-shock message. You reassess the ABCs. You can now feel your spouse's pulse, but your spouse is not breathing. What should you do next? Continue shocking? Start chest compressions? Start rescue breathing? Place victim in the recovery position?

What is your answer? _____

Why? _____

Case 1 — Answer

The best answer is to support the breathing with rescue breathing (1 breath every 5 seconds; 12 breaths per minute). You do not need to do chest compressions because the pulse has returned. You should not place a victim in the recovery position unless he or she has both a pulse and adequate breathing. Continue rescue breathing until your spouse breathes adequately on his or her own or EMS personnel arrive. You should also check your spouse's pulse periodically to confirm that cardiac arrest did not recur.

CASE 2: CARDIAC ARREST AT A SWIMMING POOL

A 52-year-old woman with a history of heart disease has been doing water aerobics in the community pool. Suddenly the class instructor sees her clutch her chest and gasp for air before she sinks beneath the water. Several people reach for the woman and drag her, wet and dripping, from the pool. The victim is not breathing and does not have a pulse. Another lifeguard runs to get the AED from the main lifeguard station. Should they shock her right away?

What is your answer? _____

Why? _____

Case 2 — Answer

The best answer is *do not shock a victim who is lying in water, even as little as a wet surface.* Try to quickly move the woman to a dry surface, and dry her chest off with a towel. Shocking a victim while he or she is lying in water may cause some arcing of electric current between the electrodes or to the AED operator. This scenario is risky because rescuers are barefoot.

CASE 3: MAN WITH A MEDICATION PATCH ON THE CHEST

An 82-year-old man has collapsed in his kitchen while getting a glass of water. His wife has called 911, and now you arrive on the scene. The man has no pulse and is not breathing. After removing the man's shirt, you discover that he is wearing a nitroglycerin patch on the left side of his chest. What should you do about this patch?

What is your answer? _____

Why? _____

Case 3 — Answer

Do not place AED electrode pads over the nitroglycerin transdermal patch. If a victim has a medication patch on his or her chest, remove it and wipe the area clean before attaching the AED. Failure to do so may result in small burns to the victim's skin.

CASE 4: ELECTROCUTION OF A CHILD

You are a Heartsaver AED rescuer who arrives on the scene and finds a 6-year-old boy in cardiac arrest in the basement of a house under repair. Next to his hand is a live electric wire, which he pulled out of the wall. After assessing the boy and finding that he has no pulse, your partner begins to open the AED and turn the power on. You stop him. Why?

What is your answer? _____

Why? _____

Case 4 — Answer

The best answer is that *AEDs are not authorized for use on children younger than 8 years of age.* The computer algorithms in the AED have been tested only with adult cardiac rhythms. Children less than 8 years old often are too small to tolerate the electric current delivered by an AED for adults. Defibrillation could damage the heart muscle. A VF rhythm could be shocked into asystole, which is even worse than VF. Future AEDs may have a pediatric shock setting. Unless specifically directed otherwise by a medical authority, rescuers should verify unresponsiveness, call 911, and apply the ABCs, including CPR.

CASE 5: VICTIM LYING ON A METAL SURFACE

A 51-year-old woman collapses on a freight elevator with a metal floor. Your partner, another police officer, has noted that the victim has no pulse and is not breathing. You get the AED from the trunk of the police cruiser, open the carrying case, and start to attach the AED pads to the woman's chest. Your partner stops you. Why?

What is your answer? _____

Why? _____

Case 5 — Answer

The best answer is that *you should avoid shocking a victim who is lying on a metal surface.* You should move the victim out of the elevator to a nonmetal surface. Because all metal conducts electric current, there is a small risk of the electric charge shocking a rescuer or bystander near the patient. If you're wearing rubber-soled shoes, the risk is virtually zero. If moving the victim is difficult or time-consuming, proceed with CPR and AED use.

CASE 6: MAN WITH RETURN OF PULSE AND BREATHING AFTER 2 SHOCKS

A 68-year-old executive collapses in his office. You and two coworkers are the company's emergency responders with the AED. You follow these steps:

- You confirm unresponsiveness.
- You send one coworker to call 911 and get the AED.
- You assess the ABCs; the patient is not breathing and has no pulse.
- You tell the other coworker to start CPR.
- You operate the AED (power-attach-analyze-shock) with loud statements to "clear."

    After 2 shocks the AED screen displays *"no shock indicated,"* and the voice prompt states "check pulse." When you check the patient, you feel a strong pulse and see the victim breathe. What should you do next? (choose one)

    A. Congratulate your coworker and remove the AED.

    B. Remove the AED and place the victim in the recovery position.

    C. Leave the AED attached and carefully observe the adequacy of the breathing and strength of the pulse.

    D. Turn the AED off and resume CPR until the victim regains consciousness.

What is your answer? _____

Why? _____

Case 6 — Answer

The correct answer is C.

You should always leave the AED power ON and the electrode pads attached to the victim's chest. Wait until EMS personnel arrive and give you further instructions. In this case the victim looks as if he has been successfully converted to a regular cardiac rhythm. Leave the AED attached. Closely observe how well the victim is breathing and whether his pulse continues to be strong.

This patient may have a second cardiac arrest ("refibrillation"). With close monitoring you will be able to detect a second arrest in seconds, and with the AED electrode pads still attached you'll be prepared to immediately analyze and shock. Monitor the victim until EMS personnel arrive. You may need to place the victim in the recovery position if he continues to breathe and has a pulse but remains unconscious.

Two important things to remember from this case: once you turn on the power and attach the pads to the victim's chest, (1) *leave the AED* ON and (2) *leave the electrode pads attached* until EMS personnel or other medical authorities tell you to turn the AED off.

REVIEW QUESTIONS

1. A victim's pulse is weak but present; however, her face has turned blue and she isn't breathing. You should attach the AED pads and start the shock cycle immediately.

   true   false

2. A victim has no pulse but has weak, sporadic, gasping breaths. He or she meets the criteria for use of an AED.

   true   false

3. The criteria for initiating CPR and using an AED are (choose one)

   a. unresponsive, weak pulse, no breathing

   b. unresponsive, no pulse, weak breathing

   c. unresponsive, weak pulse, weak breathing

   d. unresponsive, no pulse, no breathing

4. The correct sequence of actions to treat a person who suddenly collapses is (choose one)

   a. call 911, verify unresponsiveness, ABCD

   b. call 911, ABCD, verify unresponsiveness

   c. verify unresponsiveness, call 911, ABCD

   d. verify unresponsiveness, ABCD, call 911

5. You and two other rescuers respond to a 50-year-old man who is unresponsive, pulseless, and not breathing. What tasks do you assign the other rescuers while you set up the AED?

   a. one calls 911 and the other does CPR

   b. both help with setting up the AED and doing CPR

   c. both do CPR

   d. both leave to get additional first responders to help

6. After 3 shocks the victim is still pulseless. What should you do next?

   a. continue shocking immediately

   b. do not shock again until EMS arrives

   c. perform CPR for 1 minute and reanalyze

   d. remove the AED and transport the victim to the emergency department

7. You attach an AED to the chest of a 43-year-old victim who is unresponsive, not breathing, and pulseless. The AED advises *"no shock."* What would you do?

   a. shock anyway

   b. perform CPR for 1 minute and reanalyze

   c. perform CPR until EMS arrives

   d. remove the AED

HOW DID YOU DO?

1. false; 2. true; 3. d; 4. c; 5. a; 6. c; 7. b

CONTENTS

5

LEARNING OBJECTIVES

1. Explain how often CPR and defibrillation restore normal heartbeat and breathing in the out-of-hospital setting.

2. Give 2 different definitions for "success" in lay rescuer resuscitation.

3. State the importance of debriefing after a resuscitation attempt.

4. Explain the role of the debriefing facilitator.

5. Note the information your instructor gave you about whom to contact after you have attempted a resuscitation or used the AED in your location.

THE HUMAN DIMENSION OF CPR: HOW OFTEN WILL CPR AND LAY RESCUER DEFIBRILLATION SUCCEED?

Since 1973 more than 40 million people have learned CPR. Many public health experts consider CPR training to be the most successful public health initiative of modern times. Millions of people have been willing to prepare themselves to take action to save the life of a fellow human being. Despite your best efforts, however, we know that the majority of times your efforts will not succeed. CPR attempts at home or in public help restart the heart and restore breathing only about 50% of the time, even in the most "successful" communities. Research tells us that training rescuers how to use an AED in citizen CPR courses will dramatically increase the number of survivors of cardiac arrest. Still, the exact degree of success is not known. The American Heart Association supports efforts to have nontraditional rescuers use AEDs through the public access defibrillation program.

Tragically even when their hearts restart, only about half of VF cardiac arrest victims admitted to the emergency department and the hospital survive and go home. This means that 3 of 4 times your CPR attempts will be unsuccessful. We think it is important to briefly discuss the range of possible emotional reactions from rescuers and witnesses to any resuscitation attempts, especially when your efforts appear to have made no difference.

. . . .

Take pride

in your skills

as a Heartsaver

AED rescuer.

. . . .

Your success will

be measured

by the fact

that you tried.

TAKE PRIDE IN YOUR SKILLS AS A HEARTSAVER AED RESCUER

You should be proud of the fact that you are learning CPR and defibrillation skills. We hope you never have to use these skills. But emergencies happen. Now you can be confident that you will be better prepared to do the right thing for your family and loved ones, your coworkers, and your neighbors. Of course these emergencies can have negative outcomes. You, the equipment, and the emergency personnel who arrive to take over care may not succeed in restoring life. Some people have a cardiac arrest simply because they have reached the end of a well-lived life. Your success will not be measured by whether a cardiac arrest victim lives or dies. Your success will be measured by the fact that you tried. Simply by taking action, making an effort, and just trying to help you will be judged a success.

STRESS REACTIONS OF RESCUERS AND WITNESSES AFTER RESUSCITATION ATTEMPTS

A cardiac arrest is a dramatic and emotional event, especially if the victim is a friend or loved one. The emergency may involve disagreeable physical details, such as bleeding, vomiting, or poor hygiene. Any emergency can be an emotional burden, especially if the rescuer is closely involved with the victim. The emergency can produce strong emotional reactions in bystanders, lay rescuers, and EMS professionals. Failed attempts at resuscitation can impose even more stress on rescuers. This stress can result in a variety of emotional reactions and physical symptoms that may last long after the original emergency. These reactions are frequent and quite normal. There is nothing wrong with the rescuer or other witnesses.

It is **common** for a person to experience emotional aftershocks when he or she has passed through an unpleasant event. Usually such stress reactions occur immediately or within the first few hours after the event. Sometimes the emotional response may occur later.

Psychologists working with professional emergency personnel have learned that rescuers may experience grief, anxiety, anger, and sometimes guilt. Typical physical reactions include difficulty sleeping, fatigue, irritability, changes in eating habits, and confusion. Many people say that they are unable to stop thinking about the event.

Remember that these reactions are **common** and **normal**. They do not mean that you are "disturbed" or "weak." Strong reactions simply indicate that this particular event had a powerful impact on you. With understanding and the support of loved ones the stress reactions usually pass quickly.

TECHNIQUES TO PREVENT AND REDUCE STRESS IN RESCUERS, FAMILIES, AND WITNESSES

Psychologists have learned that the most successful way to reduce stress after rescue efforts is very simple: *Talk about it.* Sit down with other people who witnessed the event and talk it over. EMS personnel responding to public access defibrillation sites are encouraged to offer emotional support to lay rescuers and bystanders. More formal discussions should include not only the lay rescuers but also the professional responders.

In these discussions you will be encouraged to describe what happened. Do not be frightened about "reliving" the event. It is natural and healthful to do this. Describe what went through your mind during the rescue effort. Describe how it made you feel at the time. Describe how you feel now. Be patient with yourself. Understand that most reactions will diminish within a few days. Sharing your thoughts and feelings with your companions at work, fellow rescuers, EMS personnel, friends, or clergy will either prevent stress reactions or help with your recovery.

In some locations (for example, the homes of high-risk patients or at worksites) leaders of public access defibrillation programs may establish plans for more formal discussions or debriefings after resuscitations. Such sessions have been called **"critical incident stress debriefings,"** or CISDs.

Teams of specially trained persons are available to organize and conduct these debriefings. Such persons are usually associated with EMS services, employee assistance programs, community mental health centers, or public school systems. Other sources of psychological and emotional support can be local clergy, police chaplains, fire service chaplains, or hospital and emergency department social workers. Your course instructor will tell you what is planned for critical event debriefings in your program.

Critical event debriefings are a confidential group process. The facilitator leads and encourages persons involved in a stressful situation to express their thoughts and feelings about the event. You do not have to talk during the briefing, but if you do, what you say may help and reassure others. Rescuers and witnesses to an event can express and discuss shared feelings they experienced during and after a resuscitation attempt. These may

Review and practice sessions will strengthen your skills, build your confidence, and increase the chance of an effective resuscitation effort.

CHAPTER 5

Be proud of

your new skills

as a layperson

who can perform

CPR and operate

an AED

to save a life.

be feelings of guilt, anxiety, or failure, especially if the resuscitation attempt had a negative outcome. Ideally the rescuers who were most involved in the resuscitation should be present for the debriefing. In some public access defibrillation programs, EMS personnel visit the lay rescuers who were involved in the resuscitation effort.

In some CPR courses instructors neglect this human dimension of CPR. Frequently this is because of time limitations and a full teaching agenda. The AHA encourages medical directors and Heartsaver AED Course instructors to discuss the emotional impact and stress that may follow resuscitation attempts.

PSYCHOLOGICAL BARRIERS TO ACTION

This course is preparing you to respond appropriately to a future emergency. Although you are preparing yourself by taking this course, chances are that you will never have to use your skills. Most laypeople have never been close to a victim of cardiac arrest and have seen CPR performed only on television or in the movies. Reality is quite different. During your Heartsaver AED Course and while reading this handbook, you may have had some troubling thoughts.

Here are some of the common concerns lay rescuers express about responding to sudden cardiac emergencies. *Will you really have what it takes to respond to a true emergency?* Any emergency involving a friend, family member, or loved one will produce severe emotional reactions. Parents, for example, have felt themselves paralyzed in the first few moments of an emergency in which their child is a victim. Will you be able to take action? Will you remember the steps of CPR and defibrillation?

What about the unpleasant and disagreeable aspects of doing CPR? There was a dramatic scene in the Michael Douglas movie *The Game* where an overweight, intoxicated man collapsed in front of a main character. When the young woman rushed forward to start CPR and mouth-to-mouth breathing, the unattractive stranger vomited into her face. Would you really be able to do mouth-to-mouth rescue breathing on a stranger? What if the victim is bleeding from facial injuries that occurred when he or she collapsed? Would this not pose a risk of disease for a rescuer without a CPR barrier device?

Both CPR and defibrillation require the rescuer to remove clothing from the victim's chest. Defibrillation electrodes cannot be attached unless the pads are placed directly on the skin of the chest. The rescuer must open the shirt or blouse of the cardiac arrest victim and remove the person's undergarments. Yet common courtesy and modesty inhibit many people from removing the clothing of strangers, especially in front of many other people in a public location.

Television and the cinema have made many viewers familiar with defibrillation shocks. They know to expect the "jump" and muscle contractions whenever a character yells "clear." These shocks appear painful. Can you overcome your natural tendencies to not hurt others, even in an emergency when your actions could be lifesaving?

Often friends and relatives will be at the scene of an emergency. If you respond and take action, these people will look to you to perform precisely and confidently. Yet confidence will be hard to come by at such a rare and challenging event.

It is well known that these psychological barriers hinder a quick emergency response, especially by ordinary citizens who seldom face such an event. There are no easy solutions to help overcome these psychological barriers. Your instructor will encourage you to anticipate many of the scenes described above. Practice scenarios will include role playing and rehearsals. Think through how you would respond when confronted with such a circumstance. Mental practice, even without hands-on practice, is a good technique for improving future performance.

The Heartsaver AED Course presents a package already full of information. There is little time for an in-depth discussion of psychological barriers to action. The AHA Emergency Cardiovascular Care Committee encourages you to attend routine skills review and practice sessions at least every 6 months. The required renewal interval is **every 2 years.** These sessions will strengthen your skills, build your confidence, and increase the probability of a smooth and effective resuscitation effort. Most Heartsaver AED programs will establish review sessions to help you remain focused on the task at hand — the return of spontaneous circulation and the survival of your neighbor.

Feel free to express your concerns openly after a stressful resuscitation attempt.

The most

successful way

to reduce stress

after rescue

efforts is very

simple:

Talk about it.

SUMMARY

Rapid changes in technology have given us AEDs that are simple to operate, safe to use, and effective. AEDs and innovative emergency medical leaders have opened the door for lay rescuers to perform not only CPR but also early defibrillation. Be proud of your initiative to take a CPR-AED course. Be proud of your new skills as a layperson who can operate a sophisticated medical device to save a life.

Despite all the excitement about AEDs and public access defibrillation, there are limitations to what you can do. Your efforts will not always succeed. What is important is taking action and trying to help another human being. Some people must overcome barriers to action if asked to respond to a dramatic emergency such as cardiac arrest. Many of these barriers will be reduced during the Heartsaver AED Course. Feel free to express your concerns openly during the course and the small-group sessions.

All public access defibrillation programs that follow the AHA guidelines are encouraged to be aware of the mental and emotional challenge of rescue efforts. You will have support if you ever participate in a resuscitation attempt. You may not know for several days whether the victim lives or dies. If the person you tried to resuscitate does not live, take comfort from knowing that in taking action, you did your best.

REVIEW QUESTIONS

1. Fatigue, irritability, difficulty sleeping, guilt, loss of appetite, breathlessness, muscle weakness, anxiety, and depression are all signs of
   a. heart attack
   b. impending cardiac arrest
   c. stress response
   d. heart failure

2. The process of expressing one's feelings in a group meeting after a stressful situation such as a failed cardiac arrest is commonly called
   a. critical incident stress debriefing
   b. analysis
   c. biofeedback
   d. psychological ventilation

3. What role can the emergency professionals play after a stressful event?
   a. facilitators of a debriefing process
   b. observers of debriefing process
   c. passive participants
   d. no particular role

Your efforts will not always succeed. What is important is taking action and trying to help another human being.

HOW DID YOU DO?

1. c; 2. a; 3. a

CONTENTS

6

LEARNING OBJECTIVES

After reading this section, you should be able to

- Discuss the possibility of lawsuits and legal actions in relation to the performance of CPR
- Explain the purpose of Good Samaritan laws
- List conditions in which CPR can be stopped
- Explain the purpose of advance directives
- Discuss local and state laws related to AED use

OVERVIEW

This chapter reviews several ethical and legal topics about CPR and the use of AEDs by citizens in your community. Your participation in the new Heartsaver AED Course marks you as a concerned citizen, someone willing to make the extra effort to be better prepared.

LEGAL ASPECTS OF CARDIOPULMONARY RESUSCITATION

The American Heart Association has supported community CPR training for more than 3 decades. Citizen CPR responders have helped save thousands of lives. The AHA believes that the addition of training in the use of AEDs will dramatically increase the number of survivors of cardiac arrest.

Citizens can perform emergency CPR without fear of legal action. Chest compressions and rescue breathing require direct physical contact between rescuer and victim. Often these two people are strangers. Too often the arrest victim dies. In the United States people may take legal action when they perceive damage or think that one person has harmed another, even unintentionally. Despite this legal environment, CPR remains widely used and remarkably free of legal issues and lawsuits. Although attorneys have included rescuers who performed CPR in lawsuits, no **"Good Samaritan"** has ever been found guilty of doing harm while performing CPR.

All 50 states have Good Samaritan laws that grant immunity to anyone who attempts CPR in an honest, "good faith" effort to save a life. A person is considered a Good Samaritan if

- The person is genuinely trying to help
- The help is reasonable (you cannot engage in gross misconduct, for example, doing chest compressions on someone's neck)
- The rescue effort is voluntary and not part of the person's job requirements

Your participation in the Heartsaver AED Course marks you as a concerned citizen, someone willing to make the extra effort to be prepared.

Under most Good Samaritan laws, laypeople are protected if they perform CPR even if they have had no formal training.

Unless you are employed in a profession that expects you to perform CPR as part of your job responsibilities, you are under no *legal* obligation to attempt CPR on a victim of cardiac arrest. Failure to attempt CPR when there is no danger to the rescuer and the rescuer has the ability is considered an *ethical* violation by some commentators.

When to Stop CPR

Many citizens are troubled by the thought of attempting CPR on someone who never responds. How long do you keep doing CPR in such a situation? Stories are told, for example, about passengers in an overseas commercial aircraft having a cardiac arrest when the nearest airport is hours away. How long should you perform CPR for such an unfortunate person? The AHA recommends using common sense in such unusual circumstances. The general guidelines for stopping CPR are

- The victim responds and regains an adequate pulse and useful breathing.
- A trained professional responder takes over and assumes responsibility.
- You are too exhausted to continue, or continued CPR poses a danger to the rescuer. For example, during an in-flight cardiac arrest, do not continue CPR during landings. Stop CPR, return to your seat, and fasten your seatbelt. Resume CPR as soon as possible after touching the ground.
- A medical professional tells you to stop.
- Obvious signs of death become apparent.

What About "Do Not Start" CPR?

It is possible that you will encounter a victim of cardiac arrest who previously has expressed his or her wish to forego resuscitation attempts if cardiac arrest occurs. Friends or relatives of the victim may supply this information. Medic Alert® bracelets or wallet cards are often used as a way of communicating the victim's prearrest wishes. Many states have "**Do Not Attempt Resuscitation**" (DNAR) programs. Clear expressions of the victim's wishes should always be respected. This is discussed further in a later section.

LIVING WILLS AND ADVANCE DIRECTIVES

The Patient Self-Determination Act of 1991 supports the right of a patient to make decisions about his or her medical care, including care at the end of life. An individual may express such preferences by preparing a **"living will."** The living will documents the person's wishes, providing instructions for family members, physicians, and other healthcare providers. Everyone, particularly persons entering their senior years, should prepare a living will.

Advance directives differ from living wills. Advance directives are prepared by the attending physician or other care provider rather than by the individual. Ideally the physician writes the advance directive using the patient's living will as a guide. However, advance directives are often written for patients after they are hospitalized with a terminal condition. Frequently patients are too ill to participate in the decision making. Physicians and families should talk with patients about their preferences regarding CPR in various clinical settings. For more information, contact your physician or hospital.

EMS NO-CPR PROGRAMS

A number of states have adopted **"EMS No-CPR"** programs. These programs allow patients to call 911 for emergency care and support at an end-of-life event, for example, shortness of breath, bleeding, or uncontrolled pain. At the same time patients are able to avoid unwanted resuscitation efforts. In a no-CPR program the patient, who usually has a terminal illness, signs a document requesting "no heroics" if there is a loss of pulse or if breathing stops. In some states this document allows the patient to wear a no-CPR identification bracelet. In an emergency the bracelet or other documentation signals rescuers that CPR efforts, including use of an AED, are prohibited.

If you find a person in apparent cardiac arrest (unresponsive, no pulse, not breathing) and see that he or she is wearing a no-CPR bracelet (or has some other indication of no-CPR status), respect the person's wishes. Call 911 and report the problem as a "collapsed, unresponsive person who is wearing a no-CPR bracelet." Say that you do not think CPR is indicated and that you will await the arrival of emergency personnel.

Citizen CPR responders have helped save thousands of lives.

Citizens can

perform CPR

without fear of

legal action.

No "Good

Samaritan" has

ever been found

guilty of doing

harm while

performing CPR.

LEGAL ASPECTS OF AED USE

Defibrillators, including AEDs, are restricted medical devices. Most states have health practice acts that require a physician to authorize the use of any restricted medical device. Public access defibrillation programs that make AEDs available to lay rescuers are required to have a *medical authority*. In one sense the **medical authority** *prescribes* the AED for use by the lay responder and therefore makes the use of the AED **legal.**

In the United States fear of malpractice accusations and product liability lawsuits grows larger every year. Innovative programs to bring early CPR and early defibrillation into every community have fallen under the shadow of this fear. Physicians, trainers, program directors, corporation heads, and legal counsel for many groups have often refused to support early defibrillation programs for fear of being involved in a lawsuit. Without medical authority, lay rescuers cannot use an AED. Yet physicians are extremely reluctant to support programs that place defibrillators in homes, worksites, and public places if it exposes them to legal risk. Likewise, lay rescuers, even with physician authorization, fear being sued if they try to help someone by using an AED and "something goes wrong."

To solve this problem, many states are changing existing laws and regulations. Many legislators are amending Good Samaritan laws to include the use of AEDs by lay rescuers. This means that lay rescuers will be considered Good Samaritans when they attempt CPR and defibrillation on someone in cardiac arrest. As a Good Samaritan you cannot be sued for any harm or damage that occurs during the rescue effort (except in cases of gross negligence).

In most public access defibrillation legislation, immunity from lawsuits is granted only when specific recommendations are fulfilled. These recommendations state that the rescuer must

- Have formal training in CPR and use of an AED (AHA Heartsaver AED Course or equivalent)
- Use treatment protocols such as the CPR-AED algorithm that are approved by a medical authority
- Perform routine checks and maintenance on the AED
- Notify local EMS authorities of the placement of the AED so that EMS personnel, particularly the EMS dispatch system, are aware that you are in a setting in which an AED is available
- Report actual use of the AED to EMS authorities (usually by calling 911)

During the course your instructor will briefly discuss the method of legal immunity used in your state and what you should do to report any clinical event you might be involved in. You also will need to know who the medical authority is (often the medical director of your EMS system or the medical advisor to your worksite).

SUMMARY

There has never been a lawsuit in which a lay rescuer was found **guilty** of doing harm in attempting CPR on a victim of cardiac arrest. There has never been a lawsuit in which a professional responder was found **guilty** of doing harm in using an AED on a cardiac arrest victim. Good Samaritan laws exist in every state to give immunity to lay rescuers who try to help a person experiencing a medical emergency. The lay rescuer only has to act voluntarily in a **good faith** effort to help another person. (**Good faith** means the rescuer does not have a professional duty to respond.) The rescuer's efforts must make common sense and must be reasonable. For example, a lay rescuer cannot attempt to help in a manner that exceeds his or her skills or violates training.

The right of patients to self-determination of health care means that a patient can choose not to receive CPR or resuscitation efforts. This right should be respected. To ensure this right, some people use a living will to document their wish to forego resuscitation attempts in a cardiac arrest. A number of states have established "Do Not Attempt Resuscitation," or DNAR, programs. Patients may use Medic Alert®–type bracelets or wallet cards as a means of communicating their wishes before a cardiac arrest.

Because AEDs are restricted medical devices, a licensed physician must authorize the use of AEDs. A number of states have added AED use to their Good Samaritan laws so that a lay rescuer will be immune from legal action. Such legal action is highly unlikely. So far no lawsuit related to public-responder defibrillation is known to have been filed.

The American Heart Association recommends that course instructors provide a handout that summarizes your state's laws or regulations related to layperson use of AEDs.

The victim's wishes about CPR should always be respected.

REVIEW QUESTIONS

1. Heartsaver certification is required before a rescuer can perform CPR.

   true   false

2. CPR can be stopped in all of the following circumstances **except**

   a. the victim recovers (regains pulse and breathing)

   b. another trained person takes over

   c. you have called 911 and the EMS professionals have been dispatched

   d. you are too exhausted to continue

3. AED use is often defined by

   a. state laws or regulations

   b. the Constitution

   c. individuals

   d. contracts

HOW DID YOU DO?

1. false; 2. c; 3. a

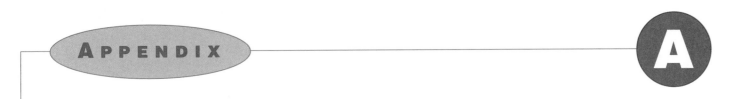

APPENDIX   **A**

HEARTSAVER AED SAMPLE COURSE AGENDA
(Slightly modified agendas may be used at specific courses.)

Introduction (instructor lecture with slides plus video)	30 minutes

- Welcome and introduction — 5 minutes
- Overview video: *EZ AED* — 10 minutes
- Overview of the Chain of Survival and automated external defibrillation — 15 minutes
  — Sudden cardiac death
  — Chain of Survival
  — Importance of early defibrillation
  — What is an AED?
  — How does an AED work?

Instruction in CPR and Relief of FBAO (videos plus instructors: "watch-then-practice")	1 hour 15 minutes

- Watch-then-practice: mouth-to-mouth breathing — 15 minutes
- Watch-then-practice: mouth-to-mask breathing — 15 minutes
- Watch-then-practice: chest compressions — 15 minutes
- Watch-then-practice: CPR (mouth-to-mask plus chest compressions) — 15 minutes
- Watch-then-practice: relief of FBAO (clearing the obstructed airway in the conscious and unconscious victim) — 15 minutes

Break — **15 minutes**

AED Instruction (instructor demonstrates — then practice)	30 minutes

- Instructor demonstrates operation and maintenance of AED — 15 minutes
  — Turning device on
  — Skin preparation
  — Location of pads
  — Pad placement
  — Analyze mode
  — Delivery of shock
  — No shock indicated
- Instructor demonstrates one-rescuer AED scenario: 1 shock; pulse and breathing return
- Participants practice Heartsaver AED algorithm (single-shock scenario) — 15 minutes

Scenario-based Practice (instructor-led hands-on)	35-45 minutes

- Practice and review: 8 critical scenarios (groups of 4; 8 rotations) — 45 minutes

Practical Evaluation (individual demonstration of practical skills; written examination)	25-40 minutes

- Practical evaluation — 20 minutes
- Written evaluation — 20 minutes

Total time: — **3½ to 4 hours**

HEARTSAVER AED RESCUER TREATMENT ALGORITHM
EMERGENCY CARDIAC CARE PENDING ARRIVAL OF EMERGENCY MEDICAL PERSONNEL
INCLUDING GUIDELINES 2000 CHANGES

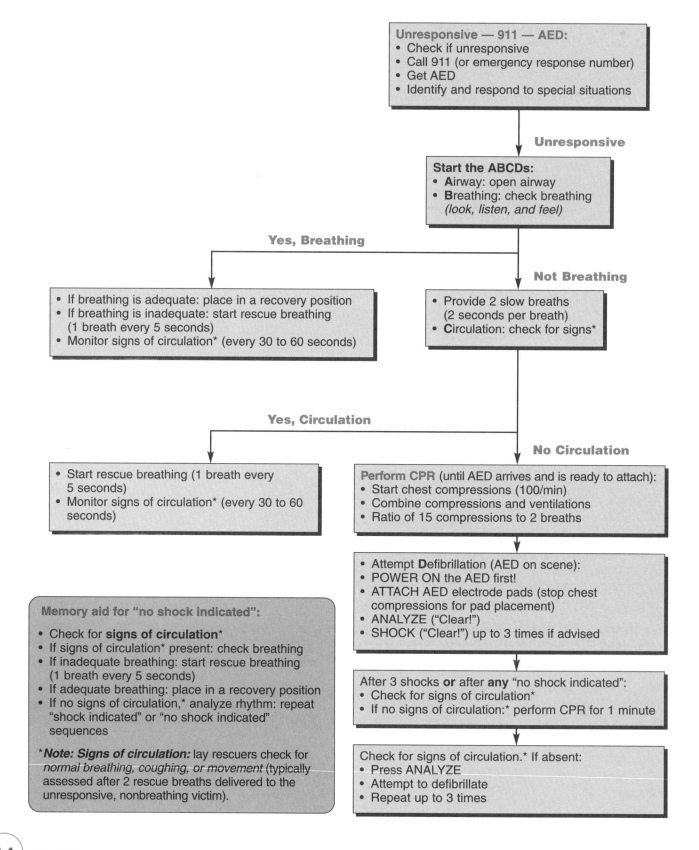

Unresponsive — 911 — AED:
- Check if unresponsive
- Call 911 (or emergency response number)
- Get AED
- Identify and respond to special situations

Unresponsive

Start the ABCDs:
- **A**irway: open airway
- **B**reathing: check breathing *(look, listen, and feel)*

Yes, Breathing

Not Breathing

- If breathing is adequate: place in a recovery position
- If breathing is inadequate: start rescue breathing (1 breath every 5 seconds)
- Monitor signs of circulation* (every 30 to 60 seconds)

- Provide 2 slow breaths (2 seconds per breath)
- **C**irculation: check for signs*

Yes, Circulation

No Circulation

- Start rescue breathing (1 breath every 5 seconds)
- Monitor signs of circulation* (every 30 to 60 seconds)

Perform CPR (until AED arrives and is ready to attach):
- Start chest compressions (100/min)
- Combine compressions and ventilations
- Ratio of 15 compressions to 2 breaths

- Attempt **D**efibrillation (AED on scene):
- POWER ON the AED first!
- ATTACH AED electrode pads (stop chest compressions for pad placement)
- ANALYZE ("Clear!")
- SHOCK ("Clear!") up to 3 times if advised

Memory aid for "no shock indicated":

- Check for **signs of circulation***
- If signs of circulation* present: check breathing
- If inadequate breathing: start rescue breathing (1 breath every 5 seconds)
- If adequate breathing: place in a recovery position
- If no signs of circulation,* analyze rhythm: repeat "shock indicated" or "no shock indicated" sequences

***Note: Signs of circulation:** lay rescuers check for normal breathing, coughing, or movement (typically assessed after 2 rescue breaths delivered to the unresponsive, nonbreathing victim).

After 3 shocks **or** after **any** "no shock indicated":
- Check for signs of circulation*
- If no signs of circulation:* perform CPR for 1 minute

Check for signs of circulation.* If absent:
- Press ANALYZE
- Attempt to defibrillate
- Repeat up to 3 times

Heatsaver AED Course
Adult 1-Rescuer CPR
Performance Criteria Reflecting
Guidelines 2000 Changes

American Heart Association®
Fighting Heart Disease and Stroke

Participant Name _____ Date _____

Performance Guidelines	Performed
1. Establish that the victim is unresponsive. Phone 911 (or other emergency response number).	
2. Open the airway (head tilt–chin lift or, if trauma is suspected, jaw thrust). Check for normal breathing (look, listen, and feel).*	
3. If normal breathing is absent, give 2 slow breaths (2 seconds per breath), ensure adequate chest rise, and allow for exhalation between breaths.	
4. Check for signs of circulation (normal breathing, coughing, or movement in response to the 2 rescue breaths). If signs of circulation are present but there is no normal breathing, provide rescue breathing (1 breath every 5 seconds, about 10 to 12 breaths per minute).	
5. If no signs of circulation are present, begin cycles of 15 chest compressions (about 100 compressions per minute) followed by 2 slow breaths.*	
6. After 4 cycles of compressions and breaths (15:2, about 1 minute), recheck for signs of circulation.* If no signs of circulation are present, continue 15:2 cycles, beginning with chest compressions. If signs of circulation return but breathing does not, continue rescue breathing (1 breath every 5 seconds, or about 10 to 12 breaths per minute).	

*If the victim is breathing or resumes normal breathing and no trauma is suspected, place in the recovery position.

Comments _____

_____

_____

_____

_____

Instructor _____

Circle one: Complete   Needs more practice

Heartsaver AED Course
Adult 2-Rescuer CPR
Performance Criteria Reflecting
Guidelines 2000 Changes

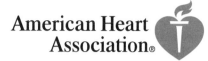

American Heart
Association®

Fighting Heart Disease and Stroke

Participant Name _____ Date _____

Performance Guidelines	Performed

1. Establish that victim is unresponsive. One rescuer should first phone 911 (or other emergency response number).

Rescuer 1

2. Open the airway (head tilt–chin lift or, if trauma is suspected, jaw thrust). Check for normal breathing (look, listen, and feel).*

3. If normal breathing is absent, give 2 slow breaths (2 seconds per breath), ensure adequate chest rise, and allow for exhalation between breaths.

4. Check for signs of circulation (normal breathing, coughing, or movement in response to the 2 rescue breaths). If signs of circulation are present but there is no normal breathing, provide rescue breathing (1 breath every 5 seconds, about 10 to 12 breaths per minute).

Rescuer 2

5. If no signs of circulation are present, begin cycles of 15 chest compressions (rate of about 100 compressions per minute) followed by 2 slow breaths by rescuer 1.*

6. After 4 cycles of compressions and breaths (15:2, about 1 minute), rescuer 1 provides 2 breaths and rechecks for signs of circulation.* If no signs of circulation are present, continue 15:2 cycles of compressions and ventilations, beginning with chest compressions, until more skilled rescuers (with an AED) arrive.

*If the victim is breathing or resumes normal breathing and no trauma is suspected, place in the recovery position.

Comments _____

_____

_____

Instructor _____

Circle one: Complete   Needs more practice

Heartsaver AED Course
Adult FBAO in Responsive Victim
(and Responsive Victim Who Becomes Unresponsive)
Performance Criteria Reflecting
Guidelines 2000 Changes

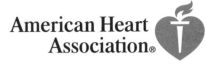

American Heart
Association®

Fighting Heart Disease and Stroke

Participant Name _____ Date _____

Performance Guidelines Performed	
1. Ask "Are you choking?" If yes, ask "Can you speak?" If no, tell the victim you are going to help.	
2. Give abdominal thrusts (chest thrusts for victim who is pregnant or obese). Avoid pressing on the bottom of the breastbone (xiphoid).	
3. Repeat thrusts until foreign body is expelled (obstruction relieved) or victim becomes unresponsive.	

Adult Foreign-Body Airway Obstruction —
Victim Becomes Unresponsive
The following is for clarification only.

4. Phone 911 or other emergency response number (or send someone to do it). Return to the victim.	
5. Attempt CPR (each time you open the airway, look for a foreign object in the mouth; if you see it, remove it).	

Comments _____

_____

_____

Instructor _____

Circle one: Complete   Needs more practice

Heartsaver AED Course
Provider CPR and AED
Performance Criteria Reflecting
Guidelines 2000 Changes

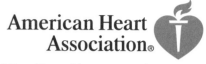

American Heart
Association®

Fighting Heart Disease and Stroke

Participant Name _____ Date _____

Performance		
CPR Skills	**Satisfactory**	**Remediate**
1. Establish unresponsiveness — direct coworker to call 911 and get the AED.		
2. Open airway (head tilt–chin lift or jaw thrust) — check breathing (look, listen, and feel).		
3. If no breathing, give 2 slow breaths (**2 seconds per breath**) that cause the chest to rise.		
4. Check **signs of circulation (no signs of circulation).** Start chest compressions (ratio of 15 to 2 breaths at **100** compressions per minute).		
AED Skills (AED arrives after 2 cycles of CPR)	**Satisfactory**	**Remediate**
5. Place the AED next to the victim's left ear; start time-to–first shock clock. POWER ON the AED.		
6. ATTACH pads in proper positions (as pictured on each of the AED electrodes, sternum, and apex).		
7. Clear victim and press ANALYZE (if present). (AED advises shock and charges.)		
8. Clear victim and press SHOCK button. End time-to–first shock clock. (May repeat 1 to 2 more analyze-shock cycles. End when AED gives *"no shock indicated"* message.)		
9. Check **signs of circulation (signs of circulation present).**		
10. Continue to check breathing and **signs of circulation** until EMS arrives. (Use of recovery position acceptable. Leave AED attached.)		
Critical Actions	**Satisfactory**	**Remediate**
• Assess responsiveness.		
• Call 911; get the AED.		
• Open the airway.		
• Provide 2 breaths (must cause the chest to rise).		
• Check **signs of circulation.**		
• Begin chest compressions (must have proper hand placement).		
• POWER ON the AED.		
• ATTACH pads to patient's bare chest in proper location.		
• Clear victim before ANALYZE and SHOCK (avoid contact with victim).		
• Check breathing and **signs of circulation** after *"no shock indicated"* message.		
• Time from start to first shock is less than 90 seconds.		

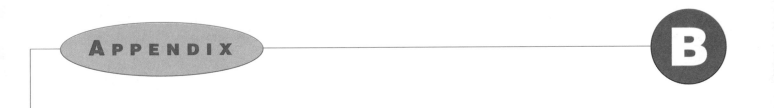

GLOSSARY OF TERMS

Algorithm — (1) A visual learning aid that teaches how to make decisions in emergencies. Using a branching, tree-like format, algorithms display conditions, treatment options, and points where decisions must be made.

(2) The process that computer chips in AEDs follow as they analyze the heart rhythm for presence or absence of a shockable rhythm (ventricular fibrillation or pulseless ventricular tachycardia).

Angina — A condition in which the heart muscle receives an insufficient blood supply, causing temporary pain in the chest and often in the left arm and shoulder, usually during physical activity or when the patient is emotionally upset.

Artery — Blood vessel that carries blood away from the heart to the various parts of the body.

Automated External Defibrillator (AED) — A restricted medical device that can assess the cardiac rhythm and determine if a shockable rhythm is present. When powered ON, the AED analyzes the rhythm and "advises" the operator to press the SHOCK control if a shockable rhythm is detected.

Barrier Devices — Plastic devices that allow a rescuer to provide rescue breathing without touching the victim's mouth or nose. They cover the victim's mouth and nose. There are 2 types: *face shields*, which are flexible and mold closely to the face, and *face masks*, which are rigid plastic and increase the distance between the victim and the rescuer.

Blood Pressure — The force of pressure exerted by the heart in pumping blood; the pressure of blood in the arteries.

Cardiopulmonary Resuscitation (CPR) — A series of actions that include assessment of breathing, rescue breathing, assessment of a pulse, and chest compressions. These actions keep oxygen-rich blood flowing to the brain until defibrillation and advanced life support can be started.

Cardiovascular — Pertaining to the heart and blood vessels, including the major blood vessels that supply blood to the brain.

Circulatory System — The heart and blood vessels (arteries, veins, and capillaries).

Coronary Arteries — Arteries arising from the aorta, circling the surface of the heart, and conducting blood to the heart muscle.

Coronary Care Unit (CCU) — An in-hospital specialized facility or emergency mobile unit equipped with monitoring devices, staffed with trained personnel, and designed to treat coronary patients.

Coronary Occlusion — An obstruction or narrowing of one of the coronary arteries that hinders or completely blocks blood flow to part of the heart muscle. See **Heart Attack.**

Coronary Thrombosis — Formation of a clot in one of the arteries that conduct blood to the heart muscle. Also called *coronary occlusion.*

Defibrillator — A restricted medical device that supplies an electric current to the heart to treat ventricular fibrillation. The current is delivered through either adhesive electrode pads that attach to the chest or hand-held metal paddles. Defibrillators can be either automated or manual.

Heart Attack — A nonspecific term usually referring to complete blockage of a diseased coronary artery by a blood clot, resulting in the death of the heart muscle supplied by that artery. *Myocardial infarction* is a more specific term for what is usually meant by *heart attack.*

High Blood Pressure (Hypertension) — Persistent elevation of blood pressure above the normal range.

Myocardial Infarction — See **Heart Attack.**

Myocardium — Heart muscle.

Nitroglycerin — Drug that causes dilation of blood vessels; often used in the treatment of angina.

Occluded Artery — One in which blood flow has been impaired by a blockage.

Pulmonary — Pertaining to the lungs.

Stroke — A sudden onset of weakness or paralysis on one side of the body (such as the hand, arm, or leg) caused by an insufficient supply of blood to part of the brain. A stroke can also affect balance, coordination, speech, or vision. Older terms for stroke are *apoplexy, cerebrovascular accident*, and *cerebral vascular accident.*

Vascular — Pertaining to the blood vessels.

Vein — Any one of a series of vessels of the cardiovascular system that carry blood from various parts of the body back to the heart.

Ventricular Fibrillation (VF) — A chaotic, uncoordinated quivering of the cardiac muscle that prevents effective cardiac contractions. VF causes cardiac arrest; biological death follows within minutes if VF is not defibrillated. VF can be removed only by "stunning" the heart with a strong electric shock (defibrillation).

APPENDIX

C

FREQUENTLY ASKED QUESTIONS ABOUT CPR

1. Can rescuers catch AIDS or hepatitis or other diseases during CPR?

It is extremely unlikely that a rescuer will become infected with either the AIDS or hepatitis virus as a result of doing mouth-to-mouth breathing or touching the victim. After more than 35 years of performing mouth-to-mouth breathing, there has never been a documented case of AIDS or hepatitis transmitted to a rescuer. You can use a face mask or a face shield as a barrier device. These devices are placed over the victim's mouth and nose to help block viruses and bacteria.

More important, about 70% to 80% of respiratory and cardiac arrests occur in the home, where the rescuer usually knows the victim and knows about the victim's health. A primary reason to learn CPR is for the benefit of your family and friends.

2. What are some possible hazards of CPR?

Poorly performed CPR can cause injuries. Follow performance guidelines at all times. Frequent manikin practice helps improve future performance. Some possible problems in performing CPR:

- Incorrect hand position for chest compression may lead to rib fractures, fractures of the end of the breastbone (xiphoid), and bruising or bleeding of the liver, lung, or spleen.
- Bouncing chest compressions may cause the rescuer's hands to move off the center of the sternum (breastbone).
- Compressing the chest too deeply may cause internal injury.
- Not compressing the sternum deeply enough may cause poor blood flow to the brain and other vital organs.
- Using breath volumes that are too great, breathing too rapidly, or not having the airway opened completely — any of these may cause you to blow large amounts of air into the stomach and cause stomach stretching (gastric distention).
- Gastric distention increases the chances the victim will vomit and may decrease the effectiveness of ventilation.

3. How do I open the airway of a victim who may have a neck injury, such as the victim of an automobile accident?

Jaw thrust *without* head tilt is the first step in opening the airway in a victim with suspected neck injury.

4. *What should I do if the victim vomits?*

   You should turn the victim's head and body to the side so that the victim will not choke on the vomited material. Then clear the airway by sweeping the mouth. A cloth (corner of clothing, handkerchief, etc) over your fingers can be used to sweep out the mouth. Then reposition the victim and continue CPR.

5. *How will I know if CPR is effective?*

   A second rescuer can monitor the carotid pulse (in the neck) while you do chest compressions. A good, strong carotid or brachial pulse (in the upper arm) should be present with each compression. Rescue breathing can be checked by looking for chest rise with each lung inflation. Remember, too much volume will cause stomach distention.

6. *How will I know if pulse and breathing return?*

   The return of a pulse, with or without breathing, may be dramatic or subtle. The victim may take a big gasp of air, begin moving, or even start to regain consciousness. If breathing is present, keep the airway open and regularly check pulse and breathing. Place the victim in the recovery position to maintain an open airway. If breathing is absent, perform rescue breathing 10 to 12 times per minute (once every 5 seconds) for the adult.

7. *What should I do about a "neck breather" in need of CPR?*

   Neck breathers are persons who have had their voice box (larynx) removed by surgery and have a permanent opening (stoma) that connects the airway or windpipe (trachea) directly to the skin. The opening is at the base of the front of the neck.

   To tell whether the victim's breathing has returned, place your ear over the opening in the neck. If rescue breathing is required, do direct mouth-to-stoma rescue breathing. For more information, contact the International Association of Laryngectomees, % the American Cancer Society, 1599 Clifton Rd. NE, Atlanta, GA 30329.

8. *If a victim is found on a bed, should I move him or her to the floor so that I have a hard surface under the victim's spine?*

   Victims receiving CPR should be moved to a firm surface. Make sure that the head and neck are supported and not left to dangle. If you are alone and cannot move the victim, leave the victim on the bed and find something flat and firm to slide under the back to provide a hard surface.

9. **What do I do for an adult who I think may be having a heart attack?**

First have the victim rest quietly and calmly. Both angina (severe pain around the heart) and heart attack are caused by too little oxygen-rich blood to the heart muscle. So keep activity to a minimum. If chest discomfort lasts more than a few minutes, the most important thing to do is activate the EMS system. (Phone First!)

10. **If I find a victim and I am alone, should I telephone for help first or should I immediately begin CPR?**

For the adult victim, phone first and then begin CPR. If you have access to an AED through a public access defibrillation program, first call 911, get the AED, and return to the patient. Provide CPR and use the AED as you learned in Heartsaver AED training. Continue until EMS professionals arrive. The sooner EMS arrives, the better the chance for survival of the adult because of the special skills of EMS personnel and devices carried by EMS units. (Phone First!)

Children have respiratory arrests more often than cardiac arrests. So for a child, begin CPR first. If after about 1 minute the child has not regained spontaneous pulse and breathing, take the least time possible and phone for help. (Phone Fast!)

11. **What should I do if the victim is wearing dentures?**

Leave the dentures in place if possible. This will help you make an airtight seal around the victim's mouth. Remove the dentures only if they are so loose or ill-fitting that they get in your way or obstruct the victim's airway.

12. **What should I do to prevent stomach swelling (gastric distention)?**

Distention of the stomach (air getting into the stomach) is most likely to occur if you blow too hard with rescue breathing or if the airway is partially obstructed. So control the force and speed of rescue breaths. Breathe slowly into the victim for 1½ to 2 seconds each time, and check that you do not continue to blow in after the chest rises.

13. **What if the victim of complete airway obstruction is pregnant or very obese?**

Treat the pregnant or obese victim of choking the same way as any other victim — unless it is impossible to perform safe or effective abdominal thrusts because the pregnancy is advanced or the obesity is extreme. In these cases, perform chest thrusts instead of abdominal thrusts. But perform these chest thrusts from the side of the unconscious victim.

14. How will I know when to start the obstructed airway sequence in a conscious choking victim?

With good air exchange the victim can cough forcefully, although frequently the victim wheezes between coughs. As long as good air exchange continues, encourage the victim to keep coughing and breathing. At this point do not interfere with the victim's attempts to expel the foreign body.

With complete airway obstruction, the victim is unable to speak, breathe, or cough. The victim also may clutch his or her neck (universal distress signal). If the victim cannot speak, begin the obstructed airway sequence.

15. Should I handle a drowning victim differently from any other victim?

Handle drowning victims exactly as you would any other victim. If rescue breaths do not inflate the chest, begin the obstructed airway sequence.

- Reposition the head and attempt rescue breathing.
- If still unable to give rescue breaths, straddle the thighs of the unconscious victim and give 5 abdominal thrusts (the Heimlich maneuver).
- Use tongue-jaw lift and sweep the mouth with your finger.
- Try again to give rescue breaths.

16. How long can I stop CPR to move the victim?

Do not interrupt CPR for more than a few seconds except for special situations, such as transporting the victim. If you have to move a victim up or down a stairway, perform CPR at the head or foot of the stairs. Then interrupt CPR, move quickly to the next flat area, and resume CPR.

17. How often should I review or refresh my skills in CPR?

The national ECC Committee recommends retraining at least every 2 years to refresh CPR skills. Your local AHA may recommend more frequent renewal of skills. If you are also trained in AED use through the Heartsaver AED Course, review at least every 2 years or refresh your skills according to local protocols.

APPENDIX **D**

FREQUENTLY ASKED QUESTIONS ABOUT AEDs

1. *Why does a person having a heart attack need an AED?*

   When a heart attack becomes a full cardiac arrest, the heart most often goes into uncoordinated electric activity called *fibrillation*. The heart twitches ineffectively and cannot pump blood. The AED delivers electric current to the heart muscle, momentarily *stunning* the heart, stopping all activity. This gives the heart an opportunity to resume beating effectively.

2. *What does AED stand for?*

   AED stands for *automated external defibrillator.*

3. *How does an AED work?*

   A microprocessor inside the defibrillator interprets (analyzes) the victim's heart rhythm through adhesive electrodes (some models of AEDs require you to press an ANALYZE button). The computer analyzes the heart rhythm and advises the operator whether a shock is needed. AEDs advise a shock to only ventricular fibrillation and fast ventricular tachycardia. The electric current is delivered through the victim's chest wall through adhesive electrode pads.

4. *Why is it important to call 911* **first** *when a person collapses?*

   While early defibrillation is the single most important treatment for VF cardiac arrest, other treatments are also needed. Even if there is an AED available on the scene, a victim of cardiac arrest needs effective CPR with oxygen, intravenous (IV) medicines, often endotracheal intubation, and rapid transport to an emergency department. These other links in the Chain of Survival optimize a victim's chances of survival and recovery. In addition, not every cardiac emergency is due to VF. Victims of non-VF emergencies need other skills and treatments from the EMS professionals.

5. *Will an AED always resuscitate someone in cardiac arrest?*

   The AED treats only a heart that is fibrillating. In non-VF cardiac arrests the heart does not respond to electric current but needs medications and breathing support instead. Also, AEDs are less successful when the victim has been in cardiac arrest for longer than a few minutes, especially if no CPR was provided.

6. What does CPR do if what the victim really needs is defibrillation?

CPR provides some circulation of oxygen-rich blood to the victim's heart and brain. This circulation delays both brain death and the death of heart muscle. CPR buys time until the AED can arrive and makes VF more likely to respond to defibrillation shocks.

7. Is an AED safe to use?

An AED is safe to use by anyone who has been trained to operate it. The AHA recommends that anyone who lives or works where an AED is available for use by lay rescuers participate in a Heartsaver AED Course. AEDs, in fact, are so user-friendly that untrained rescuers can generally succeed in attaching the pads, pressing ANALYZE (if required), and delivering shocks. Untrained rescuers, however, may not know when to use an AED, and they may not use an AED safely, posing some danger of electric shock to themselves and others. Also, untrained rescuers would not know how to respond to the victim when the AED prompts *"no shock indicated."* An operator needs only to follow the illustrations on the electrode pads and the control panel, and listen and follow the voice prompts (for example, "Do not touch the patient"). An AED will deliver a shock only when a shock is advised and the operator pushes the SHOCK button. This prevents a shock from being delivered accidentally.

8. Will I get zapped if I shock a victim in the rain or near water?

It is remotely possible to get shocked or to shock bystanders if there is standing water around and under the patient. Try to move the patient to a dry area and cut off wet clothing. Also be sure that the skin has been toweled off so that the electrode pads will stick to the skin. At the moment of pressing the SHOCK button you must make sure that no one, including the AED operator, touches any part of the victim.

9. *Can an AED make mistakes?*

An AED will almost never decide to shock an adult victim when the rhythm is non-VF. AEDs "miss" fine VF about 5% of the time. The internal computer uses complex analysis algorithms to determine whether to shock. If the operator has attached the AED to an adult victim who is *not breathing and pulseless* (in cardiac arrest), the AED will make the correct *"shock"* decision more than 95 times out of 100 and a correct *"no shock indicated"* decision more than 98 times out of 100. This level of accuracy is greater than the accuracy of emergency professionals.

10. *Why do you stop CPR as the electrode pads are placed and analysis occurs?*

For the AED to analyze accurately, the victim must be motionless. Sometimes there will be an agonal respiration (a gasping breath that can occur when the heart is stopped) that causes some movement. AEDs can recognize this extra *motion* and indicate "motion detected" to the operator. This warns the operator to assess carefully for extra movements from the victim or from the other people at the scene.

11. *Why should a lay rescuer continue CPR after the arrival of EMS professionals?*

It is helpful to EMS professionals to be able to set up their equipment, including the defibrillator, while lay rescuers continue CPR. The EMTs will take over CPR and reconfirm that the victim is in cardiac arrest.

12. *Why does it seem that the victim goes without CPR for so long during defibrillation, and why does the AED shock so many times?*

After prescribed periods of CPR, the machine analyzes the victim's rhythm. The machine requires the victim to be motionless while it decides to shock and delivers the shock. Sometimes the victim does not change from VF to non-VF at once. These victims require multiple shocks. If repeated shocks are needed, the shocks are "stacked" in sets of 3 to increase their effectiveness.

13. *In addition to using the AED, how else might a layperson help at the scene of a sudden cardiac arrest?*

    Lay rescuers are most often going to be asked to *call 911* and *get the AED*. The lay rescuer could assemble the pocket face mask and begin providing mouth-to-mask ventilations. Responders might provide CPR or continue defibrillation if a workplace defibrillator is being used. Support and direction to the bystanders, friends, and family are appropriate. When EMS personnel arrive, the lay rescuer can provide directions and help obtain information about the patient.

14. *What actions should a CPR responder take after he or she has used an AED on a person in cardiac arrest?*

    There should be some type of debriefing for the employees or lay rescuers involved. Also, collect the *voice-rhythm-shock* record from the AED's event documentation system. The AHA recommends strongly that AEDs used in a public access or home responder setting have both rhythm and voice event documentation. AEDs can record and store (at a minimum) the following information:

    - Patient rhythm throughout the resuscitation
    - Response of the AED (*shock* versus *no shock; shockable* rhythm versus *nonshockable* rhythm)
    - Event and interval timing
    - Audio recording of the voices and actions recorded at the scene of a cardiac arrest

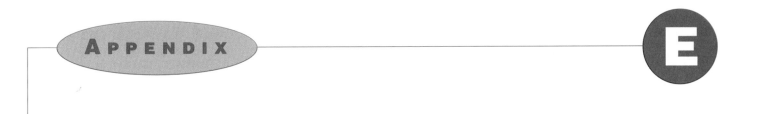

SELF-TEST QUESTIONS

Please take the following self-test. If you are unsure of the answer, take the time to review the material on the pages listed below the item.

1. *Before you try to resuscitate a victim by performing CPR, you should confirm*

   a. brain damage
   b. dilated pupils
   c. unresponsiveness and absence of breathing and pulse
   d. shallow breathing

   Answer, pp. 2.3-2.5, 4.4, 4.7

2. *The most common cause of airway obstruction in the unconscious victim is*

   a. food
   b. tongue
   c. mucus
   d. dentures

   Answer, p. 2.5

3. *The first thing that should be done for a collapsed victim of illness or accident is*

   a. examine the victim's mouth for foreign bodies
   b. determine unresponsiveness
   c. perform the Heimlich maneuver
   d. open the airway

   Answer, pp. 2.3, 4.5

4. *If the airway seems obstructed after the first attempt to give rescue breaths to an unconscious victim, you should*

   a. reposition the head and attempt rescue breaths again
   b. begin chest compressions
   c. go on to check the pulse
   d. check for foreign-body airway obstruction

   Answer, p. 2.12

5. *The method used for opening the airway is*

   a. head tilt with chin lift
   b. turning the head to one side
   c. striking the victim on the back
   d. wiping out the mouth and throat

   Answer, pp. 2.4, 2.5

6. **You can tell if an unconscious victim is breathing by**

   a. checking if the pupils of the eyes are dilated
   b. checking if the skin is cool and clammy
   c. checking the pulse
   d. looking, listening, and feeling for air movement

   Answer, pp. 2.4, 2.6

7. **If breathing seems absent after opening the airway, you should**

   a. begin chest compressions
   b. determine pulselessness
   c. check pupils
   d. give 2 rescue breaths

   Answer, pp. 2.4, 4.4, 4.5, 4.9

8. **Gastric distention (swelling of the stomach) during CPR is caused by**

   a. rapid and forceful ventilation
   b. inadequate exhalation by the unconscious victim
   c. excessive fluids in the stomach
   d. too much chest compression force

   Answer, pp. 2.6, C.5

9. **To perform chest compressions on an adult, you place one hand on top of the other with the heel of the lower hand pressing the breastbone at**

   a. the upper end
   b. the nipple line
   c. the clavicle
   d. the tip

   Answer, p. 2.7

10. **To determine if there is an obstructed airway in a conscious victim, you should**

    a. ask the victim, "Are you choking?"
    b. shake the victim
    c. reposition the victim
    d. perform abdominal thrusts

    Answer, p. 2.11

11. *To perform the Heimlich maneuver on an unconscious victim, you should*

    a. stand behind the victim with your hands grasping the waist
    b. kneel beside the victim's chest
    c. kneel beside the victim's feet
    d. straddle the victim at thigh level

    Answer, p. 2.12

12. *If a victim is coughing forcefully with a partial airway obstruction, you should*

    a. check the pulse
    b. give abdominal thrusts
    c. sweep out the mouth
    d. not interfere

    Answer, p. 2.11

13. *Foreign-body airway obstruction in the adult usually develops during*

    a. sleep
    b. eating
    c. a heart attack
    d. exercise

    Answer, pp. 1.12, 2.10

14. *When you arrive at the side of the victim, you should place the AED near*

    a. the right foot
    b. the left ear
    c. the left abdomen
    d. the right abdomen

    Answer, pp. 3.4, 3.6, 4.9

15. *One AED pad is placed on the right chest above the right nipple, below the right collarbone and to the right of the breastbone. Where is the other one placed?*

    a. over the left nipple
    b. below the left collarbone
    c. 1 inch to the left of the breastbone
    d. several inches below the left armpit

    Answer, pp. 3.7, 3.8

16. *Immediately after applying the AED pads you should*

    a. clear the bystanders and ANALYZE
    b. recheck the pulse
    c. recheck breathing
    d. push the SHOCK button

    Answer, pp. 3.8, 4.6

17. *If you use the AED to shock a victim and then receive a "no shock indicated" message, you should immediately*

    a. defibrillate
    b. check the pulse
    c. perform CPR
    d. press the ANALYZE button

    Answer, pp. 3.9, 4.6, 4.7

18. *You use the AED and deliver a shock. On the next analysis you see a "no shock indicated" message. You immediately check the carotid pulse (absent), open the airway, and look, listen, and feel for breathing (absent). Next you should*

    a. defibrillate immediately
    b. remove the AED and wait for EMS
    c. resume CPR
    d. press the ANALYZE button again

    Answer, p. 3.10

19. *You use the AED and deliver a shock. There is a "no shock indicated" message. There is a pulse and adequate breathing. You should*

    a. leave the AED attached and monitor pulse and breathing
    b. detach the AED and wait for EMS
    c. perform CPR for 1 minute and reanalyze
    d. press the ANALYZE button again

    Answer, p. 3.9

20. *You use the AED, shock the victim, and then receive a "no shock indicated" message. There is a pulse but no breathing. You should*

    a. provide rescue breathing
    b. detach the AED and wait for EMS
    c. perform CPR for 1 minute and reanalyze
    d. press the ANALYZE button again

    Answer, pp. 3.10, 4.6, 4.7